Understanding and Managing Overactive Children

A Guide for Parents and Teachers

DON H. FONTENELLE, Ph.D.

Published by

FRONT ROW EXPERIENCE
540 Discovery Bay Blvd.
Byron, CA 94514

Library of Congress Cataloging in Publication Data

Fontenelle, Don   (date).
   Understanding and managing overactive children.

   (Special education series)
   "A Spectrum Book."
   Bibliography: p.
   Includes index.
      1. Hyperactive children—Education—Handbooks,
manuals, etc.   I. Title.   II. Series.
LC4711.F66   1983   371.93   82-15010
ISBN 0-915256-21-5

To Carla, Jason, and Alan:
They have made my life happier and easier.

ISBN 0-915256-21-5

ABOUT THE AUTHOR

Don H. Fontenelle, Ph.D., has devoted most of his professional career to working with children and their parents. His efforts are directed to providing parents with a better understanding of their children and the ways to deal with their children's behavior. His workshops have been widely accepted and praised for the results that are accomplished.

Dr. Fontenelle received his Ph.D. degree in Clinical Psychology from Oklahoma State University and is currently the Director of the St. Bernard Developmental Center, a private agency providing a variety of psycho-educational services to children, adolescents, and their families. He has served as consultant for a number of children's programs in the metropolitan New Orleans area. A partial list of these agencies includes the Cerebral Palsy Center, Irish Channel Crisis School, St. Bernard Group Home for Boys, Kingsley House Nursery School Parent Training Program, Raintree House Foster Parent Training Program, and Departments of Special Education in the St. Bernard, Jefferson and Plaquemines Parish Public School Systems. He has also conducted convention workshops and inservice training sessions for teachers and staffs of agencies that are involved with managing children on a daily basis.

Dr. Fontenelle has authored a book for parents, HOW TO LIVE WITH YOUR CHILDREN (Almar Press). He has also coauthored with Mallary Collins, M.Ed., a book for teachers, CHANGING STUDENT BEHAVIORS (Schenkman Publishing Co.).

CONTENTS

FOREWORD

The level of motor activity among children varies greatly. For a personal demonstration of the diversity of this and related characteristics, such as attentional focusing and control of impulse, arrange an observational visit to a classroom of elementary-age students. Some appear quietly absorbed in their work; others are wiggly and occasionally distracted but generally centering on and accomplishing the task at hand; a few are in constant motion, attending to everything in the room except the assigned activity.

The disorganization of behavior in the last group is not limited to the classroom, but is duplicated in all areas of the child's life regardless of the situation or environment. The overactive child is the focus of a great deal of negative attention, not only from adults but from other children as well. Thus, both social and academic learning is compromised by his or her overactivity and related symptoms, which impede progress in total life adjustment.

Chronic overactivity signals a need for further investigation. Parents should arrange for a comprehensive diagnostic evaluation of the child so an appropriate plan of management can prevent serious consequences.

Child rearing is tough work, even under the best of circumstances. If a child is overactive, the added stress can disrupt all components of family life and soon exhaust domestic resources.

Child rearing is costly. The estimated financial outlay for raising a child to age eighteen is now approaching a quarter of a million dollars. Such an investment needs to be protected.

Child rearing is a kaleidoscopic process that alters with each new generation. Some time-honored principles become impossible to follow in the changing structure of family life. Many young parents are on their own, distant from their own families, who might provide the wisdom of experience and the warmth of emotional support.

Solid contemporary principles of child management that are easy to understand and put to immediate use are difficult to find. The book you are reading is an exception. Dr. Fontenelle has developed a well-organized, comprehensive child management handbook for parents of overactive children.

It is timely, tangible, and on target.

Sam D. Clements, Ph.D.

Professor, Department of Psychiatry
and Behavioral Sciences
University of Arkansas for Medical Science
Little Rock, Arkansas

PREFACE

For most of my professional career I have been seeing children for a variety of behavioral, emotional, and school-related problems. Psychoeducational specialists at the St. Bernard Developmental Center diagnose and treat children's difficulties. Diagnosis is accomplished through testing and interviewing. Treatment includes individual or group therapy with the child, but it focuses primarily on providing the parents with effective methods to manage their child's behavior. Individual sessions for the parents on techniques of child management, workshops to provide parents with more effective methods to deal with their child on a daily basis, and reading materials communicate to the parents an understanding of the problem and how to treat it in the family environment. By doing this, the parents become the child's "therapist" at home and the child can be involved in "treatment" full-time. When parents are significantly involved in their child's treatment, the probability of success greatly increases.

Overactivity or hyperactivity is a very common problem in children and a major concern for many families, because the child either is difficult to manage at home or is having trouble in school. However, not much is written for parents in this area. Almost all the books on overactivity/hyperactivity are written for professionals and are not easily understood by the average parent. In addition, many parents who come to me with children already diagnosed as overactive or hyperactive have only a vague understanding of their child's behavior. Usually when I ask them, "Has anybody ever explained to you what hyperactivity means?" the answer is "No." When the answer is "Yes," their explanation is often inaccurate (e.g., he's nervous, she has a lot of energy) or superficial.

This book was written to give parents of overactive children a better understanding of the possible causes of their child's behavior and, most important, how to deal with their child. It is written from a practical standpoint. Presenting concepts in words that we use every day. I hope this book will give you a better understanding of your child's behavior and make it easier to manage and relate to him or her on a daily basis. Although some of the methods presented here are not consistent with my own philosophy, I have attempted to describe every alternative available today to give you the widest possible choice of approaches to your child's overactive behaviors.

ACKNOWLEDGMENTS

This book is based on my experience helping parents manage their children's behavior and is the result of many learning situations. I am thankful to numerous parents of overactive children for what they have taught me. I am grateful to Lendon Smith, M.D., Barbara Miller, M.S., and Carolyn Wheat, M.Ed., for the information they provided. Dr. Smith supplied some of the information in and reviewed the chapter of diet and nutrition. Ms. Miller, gifted and talented coordinator for the Jefferson Parish public school system, and Ms. Wheat, teacher of the gifted and talented in the St. Bernard Parish public school system supplied characterizations of overactive children with high levels of intelligence. Mallary Collins, M.Ed., an educational consultant at our center, has given me a great deal of help, information, and assistance, for which I will be forever grateful. Because this book was written at home, my wife, Carla, played a large part in its completion. If she had not entertained our boys, Jason and Alan, I might still be working on this book.

I
OVERACTIVITY DEFINED

chapter one
CHARACTERISTICS OF OVERACTIVITY

How active should a child be? How restless, distractible, talkative, stubborn? What is normal behavior? Generally, *normal behavior* is that which does not interfere with a child's ability to cope with the environment or "get along" with others.

NORMAL OR OVERACTIVE BEHAVIOR?

It is relatively easy to find a child development book that will tell you at what age a child should walk, talk, get his or her first tooth, and so on. Other books will tell you what behaviors to expect at certain ages (e.g., the "terrible twos"). But what is a normal amount of sassiness, activity, distractibility, and ability to concentrate? When is an attention span short? How much should a child fidget or be restless? What is the difference between being "all boy" and being overactive? The answers to these questions are difficult to find. Almost all children, at some time or other, show overactive behaviors. Therefore, when trying to decide what is normal or what is the average amount of behavior to expect from a child, several things should be considered.

EVALUATE FREQUENCY

All children whine, have temper tantrums, show periods of stubbornness, or squirm. To determine if these behaviors should concern you, you must look at how frequently they occur. In a child who has a temper tantrum once a month or cannot sit still through some TV programs, these behaviors may not be of concern. But if the temper tantrums occur four times a day or the child cannot be still for any TV shows, even the cartoons, you need to look at the behavior more closely. The more frequently overactive behavior is seen, and the more it deviates from the average, the greater concern it should be.

COMPARE WITH PEER GROUPS

I am the last person to say you should "keep up with the Jones." But in determining what is normal to expect from your child, you have to look at the child's peer group and consider the behavior, activity level, ability to concentrate, and the like of his or her age mates. In other words, you have to compare your child to other children the same age.

CONSIDER INDIVIDUAL DIFFERENCES

Children have different personalities and show a variety of behaviors. One child may be sensitive, another talkative, yet another shy, and so forth. Therefore, in determining if a behavior is normal, you have to consider the individual child as well. There are also family differences and expectations. For example, you may expect your child to sit still while watching TV, but I may not expect this from my children.

LISTEN TO THOSE AWARE OF CHILD BEHAVIOR

Schoolteachers, coaches, nursery-school teachers, dancing instructors usually work with children of similar ages. They are familiar with age-appropriate or normal levels of activity, ability to concentrate, distractibility, stubbornness, and so on. Although they may not be able to give reasons for certain behaviors or recommendations on how to deal with them, they are often very good at identifying unusual behaviors or actions that differ from those of the child's age group. Listen to them; if several people in these capacities tell you about your child's activity level, it should be further investigated. I see many children in third or fourth grade who have shown overactive behaviors for years. I often find that the behavior had been reported to the parents by preschool, kindergarten, first grade, and second grade teachers but had not been remedied.

SYMPTOMS OF OVERACTIVITY

Children are overactive for several different reasons, but the behaviors of concern to parents fall into two general areas.

MOTOR ACTIVITY

More than the average child in his or her age group, the overactive child fidgets or squirms when he sits, is unable to remain seated for any length of time, runs when she should be walking, goes from one thing to another, cannot remain still when watching an interesting movie or cartoon, continually gets out of his chair during meals, never stops talking—in other words, he or she is in nearly constant motion.

COGNITIVE ACTIVITY

The overactive child, when compared to other children the same age, appears impulsive and distractible, has a short attention span, acts before she thinks, has difficulty following a series of directions, forgets easily, becomes easily upset and irritated, does not profit from past experiences, daydreams, is moody, has difficulty concentrating, has a low tolerance for frustration—these characteristics indicate deficits in attention span or concentration and the ability to control feelings.

Here is a list of characteristics of overactive children, divided into six areas. Most characteristics were obtained from parents and teachers of overactive children. Keep in mind that only a few or many of the characteristics may appear in a given child.

Motor Behavior
Unusual amount of energy
Excessive activity
Restlessness
Constant motion
Fidgetiness
Movement from one thing to another
Inability to sit still during meals, TV, and so on
Inability to keep his hands to himself
Overtalkativeness
Nervousness
Clumsiness
Poor gross-motor coordination
Poor fine-motor coordination
Susceptibility to accidents

Attention and Concentration
Short attention span
Poor concentration
Tendency to daydream
Distractibility
Inattentiveness
Easily aroused boredom
Frequent changes of activities
Inability to listen to a story or take part in a table game for any length of time

Impulse Control
Tendency to act before thinking
Daredevil behavior
Low frustration tolerance
Poor planning and judgment
Inability to control self
Temper outbursts
Tendency to get upset easily
Poor foresight
Poor organization

Emotions
Unpredictability

Moodiness
Poor emotional control
Tendency for feelings to be easily hurt
Impulsiveness followed by remorse
Tendency to cry easily
Fearless
Overexcitement and more activity in stimulating situations
Difficulty coping with environmental changes
Tendency to have good and bad days
Reckless
Lack of inhibitions
Dr. Jekyll and Mr. Hyde personality
Poor self-concept

Relationships with Others
Stubbornness
Disobedience
Inability to accept correction or discipline
Defiance
Refusal to take "No" for an answer
Inability to listen
Resistance to controls by adults
Negative attitude
Sassiness
Independence
Extroverted personality
Poor peer relationships
Tendency to get into fights
Bossiness with peers
Difficulty playing with more than one or two children
Overexcitability in normal play
Bold and aggressive social behavior
Tendency to be easily led by peers
Immature behaviors

Behavior in School
Tendency to leave desk
Daydreaming
Inclination to disturb others

Makes disruptive noises
Tendency to speak out of turn
Sloppiness
Disorganization
Forgetfulness
Inability to work well alone or in groups
Tendency to work best in one-to-one situation
Failure to follow or confusion of directions
Poor conduct
Academic trouble
Poor grades
Inability to keep mind on work
Failure to complete task
Can't finish work in a reasonable amount of time
Can't stay on one task
Poor penmanship
Tendency to waste time
Difficulty retaining information

Most overactive children show some difficulty in all six areas. However, a child does not have to have characteristics in all or even many of these areas to be called overactive. It is not uncommon for a child to have more problems in one area than another. One overactive child may be able to remain at his desk all day but unable to concentrate for more than thirty seconds at a time. Another child may have good concentration but be unable to remain in one place long enough to attend to the task. A child may be overactive and get along well with her peers, and so forth. Each overactive child is an individual, who presents his or her own distinct picture.

If you still feel your child's activity level differs from the average, the next step is to contact your child's doctor or a mental health professional who specializes in children. They will be able to give you information and direction.

chapter two

CAUSES
OF OVERACTIVITY

In the majority, probably 90 percent, of the children I see for over-activity, ineffective behavior management, personality characteristics and/or hyperactivity account for overactivity. A small portion of the cases, about 10 percent, can be attributed to other causes: emotional problems or intelligence. Therefore, this book will focus on the dominant factors in overactivity and will briefly discuss the other factors.

INEFFECTIVE BEHAVIOR MANAGEMENT
AND PERSONALITY CHARACTERISTICS

When ineffective or inconsistent management techniques are used by parents or there is a lack of adequate discipline in the home, children often develop overactive behaviors. These overactive be-haviors are the result of the way the child is managed, an attitude he has developed, patterns of behavior she has learned, and/or personality characteristics. For example, some children are able to avoid unpleasant duties and responsibilities or manipulate others to have most of their needs met. Because of faulty management, other children "call the shots" at home and are in more control than their parents. These children usually determine when they go to bed, whether they take a bath, what time they come in from play, when and if they will do their homework, and so on. Others are "spoiled" in the sense that they get what they want. At home they do not listen, are stubborn, appear moody, get upset easily, do not settle down when warned.

When a lot of screaming is used to discipline children, they often do not listen and tend to show other overactive characteristics. If the parents' approach to the child is inconsistent, unpredictable, and unstructured, the probability of overactive behavior greatly increases.

Spoiling

Spoiling could just as easily be called pampering, catering to children, giving in, or a number of other verbs you might think of. Spoiled children often get their way and have their needs met. They can easily manipulate their parents to get what they want. Spoiled children are more in control than their parents. This control may involve material things (toys or candy), but more often it includes behavior—getting their own way. There usually is a lack of effective discipline or parental control. These children are allowed to "do their own thing," get what they want, and exercise a great deal of control over their environment.

Overactivity caused by these conditions is especially seen in situations where limits are placed on the child or he must do things he would prefer not to do—most often this is in school. If the child is able to call the shots at home and do what she wants, when she enters a classroom setting, where much of the required work is not fun, the child will try to avoid unpleasant tasks and do what she pleases rather than what she is supposed to do. This more often occurs in first or second grade than in kindergarten, because more structure and more demands are placed on the child in those years. He looks out of the window and daydreams, because it is more fun to do that than to listen to the teacher. She doesn't remain at her desk, because she would rather get up and walk around. He does not complete his seat work, because it requires effort and he would prefer doing something else.

Parents must be in control. Children need structure, predictability, discipline, and external controls in their environment. When spoiling occurs, structure is usually lacking and an ambiguous and unpredictable environment results for the child. Consequently, he or she may become confused, try to gain more control over the environment, or become rebellious, self-centered, demanding, and selfish. These behaviors are often seen as overactive.

Spoiling, catering to a child, giving him his way, meeting all her needs, or whatever we want to call it, should be avoided. Spoiled children often develop a self-centered approach to their environment, have problems in their peer relationships because of being "bossy," fail to develop responsibility, have difficulties at school because they "do their own thing" and do not follow the classroom procedures, become rebellious, do only what they want to. Needless to say, problems will result for most such children.

Lack of Discipline or Supervision

Children who lack discipline or supervision do their own thing because of a lack of limits placed on their behavior. These children are frequently unsupervised, whether their parent is physically present or not, or are left to discipline themselves. We often think of these children as the ones who "run the streets," but this is not always the case. I have seen many situations where the parents are present, but the children are still basically undisciplined. The overactive behaviors in these children are primarily related to the lack of behavioral limits. If they are allowed to control their behavior in one situation (i.e., at home), it stands to reason that others will have difficulty controlling them elsewhere (i.e., at school).

Pleasure Orientation

Some children who are spoiled or lack discipline develop a pleasure-oriented personality. However, other children show pleasure orientation when very young, as if they are born with these personality characteristics. Frequently, these children exhibit characteristics of overactivity and must be managed somewhat differently if they are to listen and conform.

The pleasure-oriented child is primarily concerned with satisfying his or her own needs and wishes. She is more concerned with the pleasure she derives from her behavior than with the punishment. For example, the child may know that he is not supposed to do something and will be punished, but if it involves fun, he will do it and worry about the punishment later. He starts doing what he pleases and disregards rules and responsibilities imposed by others. If you ask her to do something, no matter how difficult, and she wants to do it, it will be done.

However, if you ask her to do something, no matter how small, and she does not want to do it, look out—it will be like trying to run through a brick wall. It may look as if this child acts before she thinks, but this is not totally true. She behaves in this manner because she is more concerned with what she wants to do than with what will happen to her. Consequently, this child does not listen, appears impulsive, does what she wants, and generally shows many overactive characteristics.

These children also become very skilled con artists, very much aware of inconsistencies in the environment. They are quick to manipulate people and events to satisfy their own needs and wishes or to avoid unpleasant duties and responsibilities. Their manipulation is pleasure oriented, in the sense that they want something, but someone or something is preventing them from getting it. This child knows what he has to do to get around what is blocking him so that his needs will be fulfilled. Although he can be polite, charming, and affable when it is to his advantage, this child generally has problems with authority. Such children often are rebellious, stubborn, oppositional, and resistant.

In school a variety of problems are often seen in these children, who are usually characterized by an inability to follow classroom procedure. They may be daydreaming, inattentive, and overactive. It looks as if these children have not developed any internal control, self-discipline, or responsibility, because they do not follow classroom procedure and do what they please when they please. Needless to say, this behavior pattern produces significant problems in school.

Because of the pleasure orientation, the main method of discipline (punishment) that most parents use does not work well—often it does not work at all—with this type of child. Punishment or negative consequences, when they do work, only affect this type of child temporarily—for a few minutes, at best a few days. Suppose we have two children going to rob a bank (it could be any behavior, but this serves as a good example), and we want to stop them. The first child is thinking, "If I engage in that behavior, I might get caught and sent up the river. I won't be able to watch TV, play with my friends, see my parents." The second (pleasure-oriented) child is thinking "I'm going to get some money and buy some candy, toys, and a motorcycle." We can tell the first child, "People who rob banks are punished by being sent to jail," and this will stop the behavior. However, this consequence is meaningless to the pleasure-oriented child, because he is not concerned about what will happen to him. He is more concerned with what is in it for him—what he will get out of the behavior. In the above example, we would have to take the money out of the bank (take the pleasure away from the behavior) or make not robbing the bank more pleasurable than robbing the bank.

This type of overactivity results from an attitude the child has developed or certain personality characteristics. The child in this category daydreams and looks out of the window at school because he does not feel like listening to the teacher and would rather look at the birds or cars passing outside. He continually gets out of his desk and talks out of turn because he feels like walking around and has something to say. The majority of this child's overactive behaviors are within his or her control. Such overactivity can usually be effectively dealt with by effective techniques of child management. If not dealt with adequately, these children's overactive characteristics usually increase with age.

BEHAVIOR AND PERSONALITY CHARACTERISTICS (WHEN BEHAVIOR RESULTS FROM MANAGEMENT AND/OR PERSONALITY FACTORS)

Unlike other types of overactive children, those that fall into this category usually do not show any significant deviations in their developmental history. Their walking, talking, and other skills usually develop normally. The identifying characteristics of this group are primarily in the patterns of parent-child interactions and in personality factors.

This type of overactive child is able to concentrate and sit still when she chooses to do so or is interested in something (e.g., she may be able to sit very still and quiet for two hours watching cartoons, but cannot keep still for two minutes during her mother's favorite TV program, which she views as boring). Therefore, this child appears to have some control over his or her level of activity. If you look closely at the patterns of family interaction, it usually appears that the child is in more control than his parents. Consequently, there is a lack of consistent and effective limits on his behavior.

HYPERACTIVITY: HYPERKINETIC REACTION OF CHILDHOOD (ATTENTIONAL DEFICIT DISORDER)

Not all overactive children are hyperactive. I reserve the term *hyperactivity* to describe the behavior of children who are overactive because of a hyperkinetic reaction of childhood or *attentional deficit disorder*. This overactivity results from failure to develop adequate physical controls. This child does not complete his work in school because he cannot concentrate long enough to finish the task. She daydreams because of a short attention span and cannot follow directions because she is easily distracted. Because he does not have enough control, he cannot force himself to stay still for long periods of time and therefore fidgets, taps his pencil, and generally keeps moving. The majority of these children's overactive behaviors are beyond their control; even if they try hard to prevent them, they cannot.

This child's overactive behavior results from a developmental lag or deviation. Any two children do not develop physically at the same rates—one child may walk at ten months of age, another at twelve months. Another child may get his first tooth at five months of age, while his brother gets his first tooth at six months. Any child has hundreds of skills and abilities developing within her. Some of these skills may be slow in developing. In a hyperactive child, the center of control is not developing as fast as the rest of the body.

Figure 2-1 shows that the hyperactive child's controls are not developing as fast as his or her "motor." Because this child's overactive behavior results from a developmental lag, the level of activity usually decreases with age. As the child grows, the gap between his motor and his controls will decrease. That is, if you look

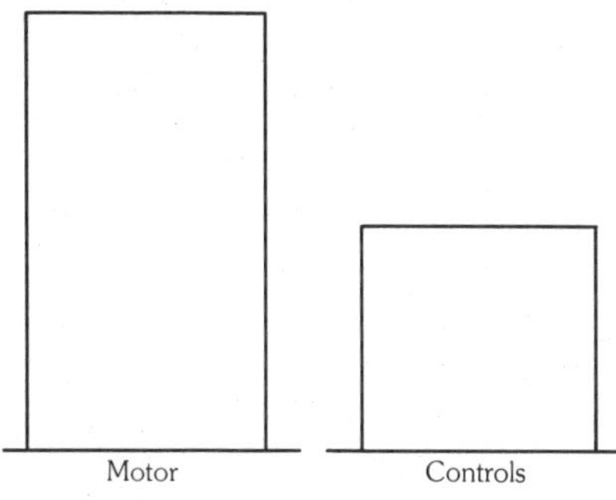

Figure 2.1. Rates of Development in Hyperactive Children

at this child at five years of age, he is less active than he was at three years of age. At seven years he shows less activity than when he was five years old, and so on. Around the time of puberty (eleven to sixteen years of age in most children), his controls catch up with his motor, his activity level seems to decrease dramatically, and his concentration and span of attention improve. This type of child will often "outgrow" his or her overactivity.

Children in this category have an intellectual potential in the average or above average range. While most of them have trouble in school because of their behavior (e.g., inability to concentrate, short span of attention, inability to sit still), some have academic problems resulting from learning disabilities and/or perceptual-motor difficulties.

Learning Disabilities

Some hyperactive children, in addition to their overactive behavioral characteristics, may have a learning disability, which will interfere with their academic performance. Most parents I work with do not know what a learning disability is. They see the learning disabled child as slow, lazy, bad, or dumb. All of these are incorrect. For a child to be classified as having a learning disability, he or she has to be average or above average in intelligence or have the potential for this level of functioning. A child may have average intelligence (like most children) or superior intelligence (smarter than 80 percent of the children his age) and not be able to read. Such children's hyperactivity may improve with treatment, but they may still show problems with their schoolwork.

A learning disabled child can learn, but not by the same

methods that most children learn. Therefore, she needs to be taught differently to acquire information and knowledge. Special education is usually needed for hyperactive children with learning disabilities.

Learning disabilities, like hyperactivity, are believed to result from developmental lags or deviations. That is, certain skills and abilities that are necessary for learning are not developing as fast as they should.

An eight year old needs numerous skills to read. To simplify this example, I will use only five areas. The child who can read has all these skills developed at the same level (see Figure 2-2). However, the learning disabled child shows uneven development in the skills necessary to read (see Figure 2-3). This child can perform some parts (Skills 1 and 4) of the reading process excellently, but she has difficulty in other areas (Skills 2, 3, and 5). When it comes time to put it all together, she cannot read. Although Skills 1 and 4 are adequate, Skill 2 may be four years below where it should be, and so on.

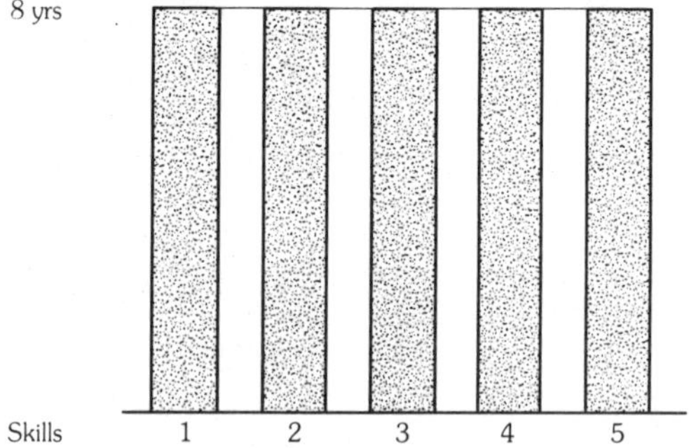

Figure 2.2. Skills Development in the Normal Child

Because we can see that these children are able to learn in many other areas (e.g., they can take their bikes apart or put together complicated models) and are not stupid, they are often classified as being lazy or having a bad attitude. In addition, their performance at school is often inconsistent. One day they get an A, the next day an F, so parents feel that the children are not trying. However, the inconsistent performance is directly related to the skill being used. For example, the schoolwork done on Monday

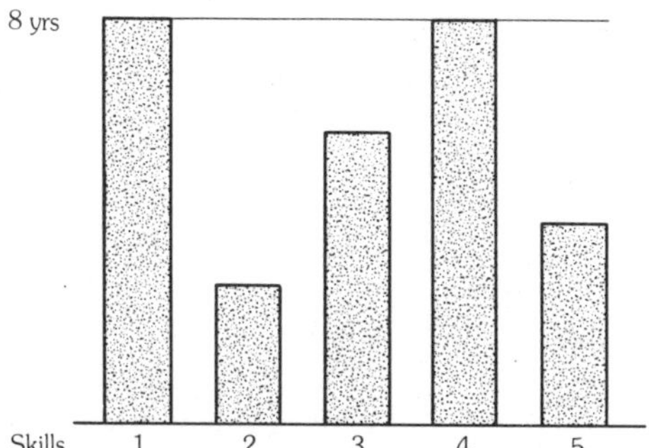

Figure 2.3. Skills Development in the Learning
Disabled Child

required Skill 1, and the child did well. On Tuesday the work was
similar but required Skill 5, and the child did poorly.

Because learning disabled children's school problems are related to developmental lags, like the reasons for the hyperactive
behavior, they usually improve with age. The gap between age and
skill development decreases. With most learning disabled children,
skills "catch up" or level out somewhere around puberty. However, if these children did not receive special education or were not
identified early in the educational process, they may have another
problem—an achievement deficit. That is, a child may be in sixth
grade and now have all the skills necessary for reading, but his
achievement or reading level may be third grade.

Learning disabilities are more common in boys than girls and
cover a wide range of learning problems. Sometimes they affect
reading, handwriting, memory, or other learning processes. For
example, a child may be able to spell *cat*, but when he sees it
written be unable to read it because he can't remember how to
pronounce the *c* or blend the sounds together.

This is only an overview of learning disabilities. An excellent
book for parents on learning disabilities is *Something's Wrong with
My Child: A Parent Book about Children with Learning Disabilities* by
Milton Brutten, Sylvia Richardson, and Charles Mangel, Harcourt,
Brace, Jovanovich, 1973.

Perceptual-Motor Difficulties
Some children classified as hyperactive show perceptual-
motor deficits, which may interfere with their schoolwork.

Visual-motor deficits and *fine-motor coordination* are other terms used to describe this problem. Basically this relates to hand-eye coordination—can a child reproduce with a pencil what she sees with her eyes?

Perceptual-motor skills improve with age. A three year old can be expected to draw a circle but usually will have trouble with a square. A five year old can usually reproduce a square, but has difficulty with a diamond. When a child shows perceptual-motor problems, his hand-eye coordination is below his chronological age. Developmental lags are considered the primary cause of this problem. As with the developmental problems that result in hyperactivity and learning disabilities, perceptual-motor skills may not be developing as fast as they should be. Problems in this area usually affect the child's handwriting skills, but in some instances they interfere with the ability to read or comprehend math. As with similar developmental problems, the child usually "outgrows" perceptual-motor deficits around the age of puberty.

Children experiencing these problems usually do not have problems with their eyes (they usually have adequate vision) or their hands (their motor development is appropriate for their age). Their problem is in how the brain processes information from the eyes and tells the hands what to do.

For these children, writing is a hard task, in fact all paper-and-pencil activities are difficult for them. Their penmanship is usually poor. They have trouble copying from the board because they leave out letters and words. Their work usually looks sloppy or careless. Because these children require a great deal of effort to perform paper-and-pencil tasks, they are "slow" at writing, often do not complete seat work, and take a long time to do a few minutes of written homework. Their writing may start off neat, but progressively it gets worse. They often reverse letters and numbers beyond the first grade, when this behavior is common to all children. Some children with perceptual-motor deficits also show gross-motor coordination problems. They tend to be poorly coordinated and clumsy. However, this is not always the case; some children with significant visual-motor deficits are excellent ball players or are very well coordinated.

DEVELOPMENTAL CHARACTERISTICS (WHEN BEHAVIOR RESULTS FROM A HYPERKINETIC REACTION)

In addition to the general characteristics of overactivity outlined in Chapter 1, children whose behavior results from a hyperkinetic reaction of childhood show other developmental patterns and traits. But some characteristics and developmental patterns of certain types of overactivity overlap. Therefore, if your child shows a few of the following signs, he is not necessarily hyperactive. You must look for patterns. Children in this category usually show a majority of the characteristics described below.

Infancy and Preschool

Hyperactive children are identified very early. As young infants, they have activity levels greater than the average infant. During their first year a large portion of these children have trouble sleeping or eating (e.g., they may not sleep all night or they often have colic). They climb out of their cribs, and their parents have little peace once such children start crawling.

When they start walking additional problems occur—they are more mobile and seem to be constantly into things. Some are able to unlock doors, cabinets, and gates and must be constantly watched to be kept from roaming the neighborhood. Others get up during the night and rearrange the kitchen cabinets. As these children grow older, it may be difficult to get them settled down to go to bed. They constantly get out of bed, talk to themselves, play with a toy, and so on. However, when you can get them to lay quietly, these children will go to sleep quite rapidly and usually sleep like a log. As they get older they sleep all night, but some tend to be restless sleepers.

Most children establish their dominant hand around the age of two. This type of overactive child often establishes hand preference later. Some continue to use both right and left hands to eat or write even after they start school.

These children sometimes show opposite reactions to medications. For example, medication for a cold or sore throat that would be expected to make one sleepy and drowsy will keep the child up all night or make him more overactive. Medications that calm down other children often produce the opposite results with this type of overactive child.

Peer problems are often present. These overactive children can play well with one child, but with more than one other child they tend to argue. Problems are more evident in group play because these children usually try to control others. They also may show immature behavior in peer interaction.

School Age

Although these children have average or above average intelligence, they often have problems in school. These problems usually are more behavioral than academic, but in the later grades the child's behavior may interfere with school performance. They tend to be impulsive, moody, and often have problems following a series of directions. The overactive behaviors in these children seem to decrease with age.

LOWER OR HIGHER THAN AVERAGE INTELLIGENCE

Although infrequently, level of intelligence appears to be related to increased levels of activity in some children. As some children approach the extremes (both high and low) of the range of intelligence, their probability of overactive behavior increases. That is, some gifted children as well as some children with relatively low intellectual functioning show increased activity levels, short attention spans, and other characteristics of overactivity. Before discussing these overactive children, I will present a general overview of intelligence.

WHAT IS INTELLIGENCE?

There is a lot of disagreement among professionals regarding this question, but we can define intelligence as a child's capability, his potential, how smart she is, his ability to learn. Intelligence, like physical characteristics, is inherited. A child is born with a certain level of intelligence and, for all practical purposes, it does not change throughout life. The child's capacity to learn is inherited primarily from parents and grandparents, but it is possible for a child to inherit characteristics from any generation of his or her family tree.

Let's look at an example of height. My mother is 4'10" and my father is 5'5", so it stands to reason that I was not going to be a basketball player. I am about 5'5", and this was set at birth. No matter what I did or how hard I tried, I would not achieve a height greater than 5'5". However, if I was sick, had an accident, or did not eat properly, I would not reach this height. Although my height conforms roughly to the height of my parents, I might have inherited this characteristic from another generation in my family tree and could have been a basketball player. Intelligence is determined in a similar way. There is a good probability that a child's intelligence will be similar to that of her parents, but it is also possible that a couple with high intelligence will have a slow child or vice versa. Intelligence is fixed at birth; you cannot get "smarter" with time, but capacity could be lowered if something interferes with physical development.

MEASUREMENT OF INTELLIGENCE

Intelligence is usually measured by a test that has been given to thousands of children of the same age. The child's score is compared to that of the other children to determine whether the child is below average, average, or above average. Individual tests, given on a one-to-one basis, yield more accurate results than tests given in a group.

One way to describe intelligence (IQ) is in terms of a child's mental age (as determined by a test) divided by chronological age, multiplied by 100.

$$\frac{\text{Mental Age}}{\text{Chronological Age}} \times 100 = \text{IQ}$$

Because some problems were encountered with this method of determining IQ, most modern tests use a *deviation IQ*, which obtains IQ by comparing statistically each child's test performance exclusively with the scores earned by children in his or her own age group.

The actual IQ number is not very important; what should be looked at is the range of a child's intelligence. The distribution and ranges of intelligence are shown in Figure 2-4.

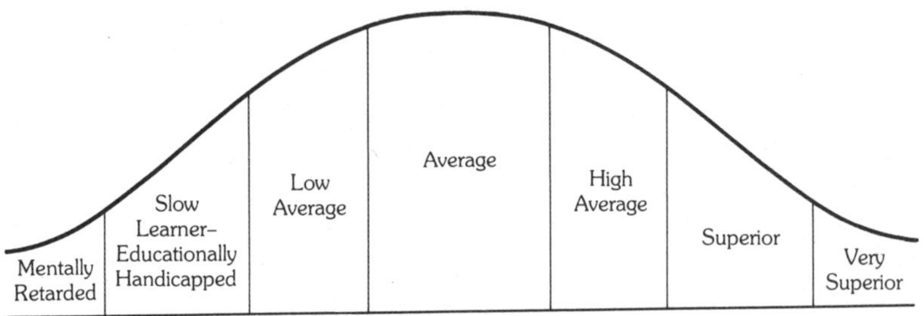

Figure 2.4. Distribution and Ranges of Intelligence

The average range of intelligence includes about 50 percent of the children in the United States. About 25 percent of children are above average and about 25 percent are below average in their ability.

OVERACTIVITY AND INTELLIGENCE

Some children on the extremes of the ranges of intelligence show overactive behaviors—those whose ability falls in the middle limits of the superior range and above or in the middle limits of the slow learner–educationally handicapped range and below. *Some*, not all, children in these ranges show increased levels of activity, distractibility, impulsiveness, and other characteristics of overactivity.

High Intelligence

Some children whose level of intelligence falls within the middle limits of the superior range of intelligence and above (IQ of approximately 125 and higher) show overactive characteristics. Approximately 7 percent to 8 percent of the total population falls within this intellectual range, and only a small portion of these show overactive characteristics. Some children in this range of ability are difficult for their parents to manage. You have to run faster to stay one step ahead of the brighter child. These children are often curious and overtalkative. They ask a lot of questions and require logical reasons for "No" or "You can't do that." They show some overactive characteristics at home, but the biggest problem they present for their parents is discipline.

Although bright, these children sometimes have problems in school. They talk out of turn, do not pay attention, do not complete seat work, refuse to do repetitive activities, and may show poor grades because of incomplete work. They may be bored, or the material presented may not be challenging enough. They refuse to write words ten times each because they already know how to spell them. They do not complete a page of addition problems because they already know how to add, and so forth. Instead of doing their work they talk, get out of their desk, make noises, draw, and show other signs of distraction.

Some of the overactive behaviors in these children come with their high level of intelligence and have to be accepted. But their behavior patterns can be changed.

Depressed Intelligence

Some children whose level of intelligence falls in the middle limits of the slow learner–educationally handicapped range and below (IQ of approximately 75 and lower) show overactive characteristics. About 7 percent to 8 percent of the total population falls within this intellectual range, and some of these children show overactive behaviors. Although a depressed level of intelligence can be inherited, it can also result from other factors. Improper nutrition, sickness of the mother (e.g., German measles), or other factors during pregnancy may interfere with adequate fetal development and produce a depressed level of intelligence or brain damage. After birth a child may experience a disease (e.g., high fever) or injury that produces brain damage and results in lower intelligence.

Some children with lowered IQs are easily distracted, impulsive, stubborn, and so on. At home they are generally difficult to manage and may be discipline problems for their parents. At school they show the typical problems—not being able to sit still, talking out of turn, having difficulties with peers—but they also are "slow" in their schoolwork and tend to have difficulty with academic studies. They may not understand the work or may be ''behind'' in their work. Consequently, some of what happens in the classroom does not make sense to them. They may daydream, talk, and show many other school-related overactive behaviors.

Because some of the overactive behaviors in these children result from brain damage, they will not change. Usually their overactive behaviors stay the same or increase with age. However, other behaviors can be modified. In the school environment special educational services may be necessary, and communication may have to be established between the parents and the school.

DEVELOPMENTAL CHARACTERISTICS (HIGH LEVELS OF INTELLIGENCE)

In addition to the general characteristics of overactivity, children with intelligence significantly above average show other developmental patterns and traits. It does not mean that a child is very intelligent if he shows a few of these signs. We look for patterns, and most gifted children show a majority of the characteristics listed below.

Infancy and Preschool

While some gifted children have slight delays in speech development, most achieve the developmental milestones early. Their accelerated development in language and understanding relationships are usually the first things noticed.

These children show early use of a large and accurate vocabulary. At an early age they use entire sentences and can reproduce a story. They are keen observers and retain a significant amount of information about things observed. They have an early interest in books, calendars, and telling time. They learn to read early and later enjoy atlases, dictionaries, and encyclopedias. These children ask many questions and show an avid interest in exploration and cause-and-effect relationships. They have a great deal of curiosity, and they generate many ideas or solutions to problems. They see many aspects of one thing (i.e., they fantasize, imagine, manipulate) and are adventurous and speculative.

These children communicate easily with others and relate well to adults. They get along better with older children than with those their own age. While these children often exhibit leadership qualities, they are sometimes aggressive, domineering, and bossy with age mates. They can amuse themselves quite well, and their solitary play often involves complicated projects or elaborate stories with many characters. They may also have imaginary playmates.

School Age

These children learn rapidly and easily but often prefer to learn by creative means rather than from an authority. Consequently, they seem to want to do their own thing in the classroom. They are easily bored with routine tasks and may refuse to complete tasks they already know. They may also cause problems in the class because they finish work faster than the other students.

These children often read independently for information and pleasure and usually perform academically at least two years above their grade level. They get absorbed in a particular task and strive to complete it. They have unusual abilities in organizing, integrating, and evaluating ideas.

In the classroom they are alert, keenly observant, quick to respond; they use much common sense and practical knowledge. They reason things out, see relationships, and comprehend meanings that other children find difficult. They ask many questions, are interested in a wide range of things, and seem to know about many things of which other children are unaware.

Although in some of these children activity level increases with age, the majority maintain the same level of activity.

DEVELOPMENTAL CHARACTERISTICS (DEPRESSED INTELLIGENCE)

In addition to the general characteristics of overactivity, children whose increased activity is related to depressed intelligence often show other characteristics and developmental patterns. If your child shows a few of the traits listed on the next page, it does not necessarily mean he or she has a low level of intellectual functioning; children with depressed intelligence usually show most of these characteristics.

Infancy and Preschool

Many of the children in this category show mild to moderate delays in the developmental milestones (e.g., walking, speech, habit training, language, and coordination). They often are unable to combine words into sentences, and they lack imagination. Their play is often simplistic. Social immaturity is present, and they tend to choose younger playmates.

School Age

The children in this category who are not identified earlier are clearly recognized when they start school, because the main characteristic of this group is difficulty with schoolwork. They may have trouble learning the alphabet, numbers, and so on. In kindergarten, and especially in first grade, the teachers communicate to the parents that these children are not ready for the next grade. These children have difficulty abstracting and dealing with complexities in the environment. If steps are not taken to alleviate school difficulties, other behavioral problems might arise (e.g., withdrawal, negativism, aggression). The activity level in these children usually stays the same as they grow, but in some instances it may increase.

EMOTIONAL PROBLEMS

Although a large number of overactive children are described as "nervous," only a very small portion of overactive behavior in children results from emotional difficulties. Only about 2 percent or 3 percent of the total child population experience significant emotional problems. Some children show significant problems at an early age regardless of the home environment, and their behavior seems to result from genetic factors. Other children experience an unpredictable, ambiguous, chaotic, or inconsistent environment, become confused, uncertain, or insecure, and start losing contact with reality. Children in either of these situations often show increased levels of activity.

If you or I say we are nervous or are experiencing emotional discomfort, we usually mean that we are fidgety, have a hard time concentrating, have a short attention span. Some overactivity seen in children is similar and results from emotional difficulties.

Children with serious behavioral problems do not necessarily have emotional problems, but the behavior of a seriously emotionally disturbed child almost always deviates from that of other children the same age. Let me first define behavioral problems and emotional difficulties. Suppose you are sitting with me in a room and a man puts a gun by my head, but you do not see this. All you can see is my behavior—I'm shaking, my voice is trembling, I start to sweat, I'm having difficulty paying attention to what you are saying, and so on. You would look at me and say, "That fellow has a problem." You would be right, but I would have more of a behavioral problem than an emotional one. My behavior would be more related to the environment than to underlying emotional difficulties. Therefore, a behavior problem can be viewed as a response to the environment; it is more superficial than an emotional difficulty. Change the environment (i.e., take the gun away from my head), and my behavior will change.

On the other hand, emotional difficulties are "deeper" or more internally based problems. For example, this man keeps putting the gun to the side of my head every hour for a few months. Soon the gunman would not have to be present for me to be a "nervous wreck" and show many problem behaviors. Now I would have emotional problems because they would be internal and more part of me than a response to the environment.

There are three general theories on how serious emotional problems develop in children. One considers genetics and heredity as major factors—the child is born this way. Another stresses environmental influences—the child's behavior is a result of what he or she has experienced. The third combines heredity and environment. In its view heredity sets the stage and the environment determines what players are used. That is, a child may inherit a predisposition for emotional difficulties but must experience certain environmental conditions for emotional problems to appear.

I favor the last explanation, but I have seen children whose history and behavior are consistent with the other two theories. For example, children from apparently "normal" and "emotionally healthy" families sometimes show emotional problems. In contrast, some children experience horrible environments (e.g., they are neglected, abused, have seriously disturbed parents) and emerge free from significant emotional problems. Others are apparently free from serious emotional disturbance until they experience a chaotic, unpredictable, changing, environment.

Only a small portion of children show emotional difficulties, and only some of these children have overactive characteristics. The psychological terms often used to describe these children's conditions are *preautism, autism, childhood psychosis, childhood schizophrenia, borderline personality,* or *severe neurosis* (e.g., excessive fears, anxieties, worries, compulsive behaviors). Most such children are identified early, usually before they enter kindergarten.

DEVELOPMENTAL CHARACTERISTICS (EMOTIONAL DIFFICULTIES)

In addition to the general characteristics of overactivity, children whose increased activity has an emotional base often show other characteristics and developmental patterns. The information presented below is based on my experience, as well as research data. A child with emotionally based overactivity usually shows a majority of these characteristics.

Infancy and Preschool

In infancy these children show two different patterns. Some are described as "too good" and never troublesome. They are very placid, passive, and undemanding. They may seem content lying quietly in bed all day. These children do not cry often; their mothers often have to base feedings on time, because these children do not cry when hungry. They do not raise their arms to be held, and they do not seem to like to be comforted. They also may show rocking behaviors when falling asleep or at other times.

The others show little active interest in the environment, but they are often described as problem or difficult babies. They often have sleep problems, cry a great deal, and fight daily routines (e.g., bathing, dressing, changing diapers). These children may also show feeding problems and may have difficulties sucking. They also are difficult to comfort, but unlike the passive infants, they may become stiff when held or actively resist their parents' physical contact. Although holding them will not generally reduce their crying and distress, some of these children will calm down when held in an unusual manner (for instance, in a stiff position on their mother's hip).

In infancy as well as throughout their early life, these children often show distinct general characteristics. They appear socially aloof and withdrawn and act as if other people are not present. They resist changes in routines and in the environment, sometimes with violent reactions. They also show an inability to play and may display specific fears.

Somewhere between two and five years of age, the problems of these children become more noticeable. Although some of these children show lags in the developmental milestones, most show difficulties in speech development. This is how most of these children are identified.

These children may not speak at the appropriate time, or if they do speak, they show definite problems. Their speech may be delayed or immature. Poor pronunciation (e.g., leaving out letters or parts of words) may be present, as well as baby talk. They may speak in meaningless or scrambled sentences, and most often their attempts at communication are unintelligible. They may confuse words (*shoe* for *suck*) or develop their own language (*bint* might mean *gum*). *Echolalia*, or parrot talk, may be present. That is, they will repeat what others say. Or these children may perseverate, say things over and over again.

Often parents or teachers of these children feel that they may have hearing problems. They often ignore sounds, do not listen or respond when spoken to, and have difficulties in voice control (e.g., they may talk loud at one time and low the next minute). While they may ignore certain sounds (e.g., a pot dropping right behind them), they may be highly sensitive to others or show violent reactions to some sounds (e.g., a vacuum cleaner or a fire engine siren).

Some children in this category reach the developmental milestones at the appropriate ages, but then experience a change in the environment or a traumatic situation and regress. For example, a child starts talking at the normal age, but gets into an auto accident or experiences a significant conflict between his parents and then stops talking. Another child may have been toilet trained for many months, but a new sibling is born or she moves to another house and starts having accidents.

Children with emotionally based overactivity may also have problems understanding things they see. In addition to being unresponsive to verbal interaction and sounds, these children sometimes do not respond to or understand gestures. Their eyes usually do not fix on one object, especially a person, but constantly scan the room, looking for movement. When an object or person is in movement, they may attend to that. In addition, they may become fixated on or fascinated with moving or whirling objects like a blender or a fan.

These children may also show unusual reactions to their other senses. They may be hypersensitive to or show little reaction to pain. They may like to rub textured materials, furs, or smooth objects. In addition, they may like to put everything in their mouths, taste things, or smell their food before they eat it.

Some overactive children with emotional problems show unusual body movements, such as rocking, head bumping, unusual walking patterns, and preoccupation with movement of their bodies or body parts, such as fingers. They also may show difficulties in fine-motor coordination.

School Age

Although three-quarters of these children are identified by age five, many of the above characteristics are also seen in the school-aged child. Some of these children have academic problems, but many do not. However, most have difficulty in peer interaction and are described by their elementary-school teachers as "loners," "in a world of their own," or "not following classroom procedures or routines."

Most of the overactivity in these children is seen from an early age and intensifies with time. At age five, these children are more active than at age three, and at seven years of age they are showing even more overactive characteristics.

Some children show overactive characteristics related to severe neurotic problems (e.g., anxiety, depression) or situational events (e.g., parental conflict, school stress, moving). Although these children do not show the early characteristics or developmental patterns described above, they usually respond to the treatment methods used to deal with children with significant emotional problems.

COMBINED CAUSES

As with most behavior, there is very seldom a clear-cut cause for overactivity. Behavior is complex and usually is the result of the interaction of several factors.

Overactivity resulting from level of intelligence and emotional difficulties is very infrequent; it accounts for less than 10 percent of increased levels of activity in children. Management difficulties or personality characteristics and hyperkinetic reactions of childhood cause the majority of overactive behavior in children. Consequently, the most frequent combined causes of overactivity arise from these two factors. For example, a child may show some signs of a hyperkinetic reaction of childhood and is, therefore, somewhat difficult to manage. Consequently, her parents may overlook some of her behaviors and give in to her to avoid a hassle, resulting in an increase in her overactivity.

Very frequently I see children who are overactive, but whose test data, developmental histories, teacher reports, and behavioral observations only give hints of a hyperkinetic reaction of childhood. That is, there are only slight to marginal signs that the child's overactive behaviors are beyond his or her control and are caused by developmental factors. Usually in these situations, problems in discipline also exist. That is, some of the child's overactive behaviors are resulting from a lack of effective, consistent, and predictable behavior management techniques.

Before any specific techniques for the management of overactivity behaviors are employed, I attempt to determine what overactive behaviors the child can and cannot control. I do this primarily by using the general techniques of behavior management discussed in Part II. Basically, I try to have the parents establish a consistent, structured, and predictable home environment and employ rewards and positive consequences as the main method of discipline.

II
GENERAL MANAGEMENT TECHNIQUES

chapter three

PROVIDING A STRUCTURED AND PREDICTABLE ENVIRONMENT

All overactive children, regardless of the reason for their increased activity, respond well to predictable and structured environments. In a fluid, inconsistent, or unpredictable environment, overactive behaviors increase. Most parents of overactive children see this often. Let's say a family is watching TV, everything is calm, and Preston is quietly playing with his cars. Then his father says, "Let's go get an ice cream." It seems as if Preston has suddenly been activated. He is energized, up and down, talking, and showing numerous overactive behaviors, as if he had been hit by a live wire. Another example is when someone drops over unexpectedly. Everything is calm, but as soon as the bell rings or the person comes in the house, the child is "bouncing off the walls." These children are reacting to a change, something new in the environment, and the fact that the environment has lost some structure and predictability.

The more structure, predictability, and consistency exist in the environment, the more overactive children will "slow down" and listen, and the greater effectiveness of discipline will be. A predictable and structured environment primarily centers around how consistent the parents are in dealing with their children and how rules are set and enforced. The following sections will provide you with some general principles and techniques with which to manage and discipline all types of overactive children on a daily basis.

ESTABLISHING CONSISTENCY

Many overactive children are described as "hardheaded," "stubborn," "not doing what they are told," or some other phrase that identifies one of their problems as not listening. One of the primary reasons for this behavior is inconsistency in their parents' approach to it. Parents often do not mean what they say or do not follow through. Although this seems like a simple concept, it is one of the main reasons why techniques tried by parents do not work. In addition, not following through produces confusion, unpredictability, and lack of structure in the environment. For some children this results in increased levels of activity.

Consistency can be viewed as the foundation of managing overactivity. By being consistent, parents increase the probability that the techniques they use will work. On the other hand, an inconsistent approach to child management almost assures failure and behavior problems.

We do not listen to adults who say one thing and do something else. So we cannot expect our children to listen to us if we behave in the same way. Let's take an example. Suppose you have a friend who continually is telling you things like "I'll come and drive you to the store tomorrow" or "I'll help you move your furniture Saturday." But he seldom follows through with anything he says. He says one thing and does something else. How would you respond to your "friend"? You would not listen to him. More important, he would not be able to control you or get you to do what he wants. He tells you to wait for him to come over on Saturday, but you go about your daily business. If you are inconsistent in your approach to your child, he or she will feel the same way about you and will respond to you the same way you responded in this example.

STATEMENTS NOT MEANT

A child is drinking a Coke on your new couch. He spills it, and you say, "Now look what you've done. You can't have any more Coke for the rest of your life."

Your child keeps running through the house and you tell him, "The next time you run, you are going to get it." He continues to run, and

after forty-nine more "runs" through the kitchen, you are still saying "The next time that happens . . ."

You tell the child, "I'm going to count to three and you better stop
doing that. One, two, two, two, two and a half, two and five-
eighths . . ." Three never comes.

You are driving across town and have your two children in the
backseat. They are picking on one another, and you are asking them
to keep still. However, their behavior intensifies. Now you are hollering. The kids start to fight, and, at the end of your rope, you say
something like, "If you don't quit that, I'm going to stop at the next
bridge and throw both of you off."

You are watching TV with your son and daughter. The boy keeps
pulling his sister's hair and aggravating her. You try to get him to
stop, but he does not respond to your pleas. Eventually you attempt
to control him by saying, "If you hit your sister one more time, I'm
going to break both of your arms."

The point is that we often say things we do not follow through or
have no intention of carrying out. We know this, but, more important, the child knows it too. Therefore, the threat does not stop the
behavior.

OVERSTATEMENTS

You are sitting down with your son trying to get him to do his
homework, but he's daydreaming, beating the pencil on the table,
and so on. Fifteen minutes of homework has lasted two hours, and
all your attempts to get it finished have failed. You are frustrated and
finally tell him, "Go to your room, you're punished for the night."
He starts crying, but goes to his room and pouts. In a few minutes he
is sticking his head out of the door and saying, "I'm sorry, I love
you, I'll be good, I'll never do it again." You start feeling sorry for
him or feeling guilty for what you have done, and two minutes later
you let him out of his room.

Your daughter has left her bike outside. The next morning you find
it and say, "Your bike is going to be stolen. I've told you many times
to bring it into the backyard. Now you can't ride it for the rest of the
month." However, in two days, she is back on her bike.

Overstatements like these are also major sources of inconsistency
in families. You get angry and make a statement you could never
keep or do not intend to keep. Or you say or do something, then

feel guilty and try to undo it. In these instances the child interprets the parent's behavior as saying, "Don't believe or listen to what I say because I don't mean it."

TURNING "NO" TO "YES" AND "YES" TO "NO"

Another way to be inconsistent is to change what you say.

> You tell a child to go take a bath, but he feels stubborn, and a hassle starts. "I don't want to. I took one last night." Nothing you say changes his mind. After thirty minutes of trying unsuccessfully to get him in the tub, you say, "OK, you don't have to take a bath tonight."

> A child is told that he will go fishing Saturday. He has been waiting for two weeks, but Friday night his father says, "I'm too busy to go fishing tomorrow. We'll go next week."

> It is about thirty minutes before supper and your six-year-old daughter comes up to you and says, "I'm hungry. Can I have a cookie?" Your response is, "No, we're going to eat in a little while, and if you eat the cookie you won't eat supper." However, she does not accept this. Each time her voice is getting louder and louder. She whines, complains about how mean you are, hits her sister, or says she would rather live with her grandparents. While all of this is going on, you are telling her to calm down, be quiet, stop whining, and so on. After about three minutes, your nerves are on end, you have burned your finger on the stove, and you are fed up with her behavior. So you give your daughter the cookie and tell her to get in the other room to eliminate the hassle and preserve your sanity.

> You take your nine year old to the department store. He has always given you trouble there, but you are hoping it will be different this time. However, as soon as you pass the toys, he grabs something and says, "I want this car." You reply with the standard answer, "No, you put that back. I don't have enough money to buy that car, and you have ten at home just like it." However, he does not put it back and as you shop he continues to tell you how much of a necessity the car is. You get everything you need and head for the checkout counter but have to wait in line. While there, your son intensifies his efforts to get the car. He really starts complaining. "You never get me a thing, and you are always buying my brother toys. You're mean." Then he really starts crying, hitting the counter, and starting to embarrass you. To shut him up you say, "I just found some money I didn't know I had. Now be quiet and I'll get you the car."

In this form of inconsistency a "no" is changed to a "yes," or a positive statement becomes negative. The environment becomes fluid, and structure and predictability are lost. Not only are we teaching our children not to listen to us when we respond in this fashion, but also we are showing them how to manipulate us. We are saying, "If I tell you something that you do not like, do this or that [have a temper tantrum, become active, whine] and I'll change my mind."

NOT CHECKING TO SEE
IF WHAT YOU SAID HAS BEEN DONE

You can also produce inconsistency by telling your child to do something and not checking to see that it has been done.

> Your child comes home from school, gets undressed, gets his snack, and says, "Can I go outside and play?" You say, "Sure, as soon as your room is straightened and everything put where it should go." He goes in his room, and you are busy in the kitchen. In about five minutes he returns and says, "I'm going outside." You say, "Did you pick up your room?" He responds positively and leaves. About an hour later you pass his room and see that nothing has been changed. You are furious but cannot locate him.

> You are sitting in the den watching TV and tell your child, "It's time to go to bed. Go brush your teeth and go to bed." She gets up, goes in the bathroom and then to her room. You ask, "Did you brush your teeth?" She says, "Yes." Later, upon entering the bathroom you see that all of the toothbrushes are dry. You now go to her room to tell her, but she is sleeping.

Overactive children are often easily distracted and "forget" to do some things. Therefore, it is important to follow up and see if the child has done what he or she was supposed to do.

CONSISTENCY FROM BOTH PARENTS

Consistency must come from both parents as a unit, in addition to individual consistency. Each parent must have similar rules and expectations for the child's behavior. You want to avoid having different rules. For example, the father lets his son jump on the furniture, but the mother doesn't. Mother allows the child to "talk back" and generally be sassy, but father does not. Father could care less about homework, but mother is concerned and makes the child do it.

Consistency also comes from the parents as a unit; they must support each other.

> A child comes up to her mother and says, "Can I make some popcorn?" She says "No." Then she asks her father and gets a positive answer. Now she's in the kitchen making the popcorn, and her mother comes in and says, "What are you doing? Didn't I tell you not to do that?" She responds with, "My dad said I could do it." Her mother storms out of the kitchen and starts a discussion with her husband that becomes an argument. In the meantime, their daughter is sitting in the kitchen eating popcorn.

> A child has been sassy all afternoon and at the dinner table he starts talking back to his father and is told, "If you do that one more time, you can't watch TV tonight." The boy continues to be sassy and his father tells him, "Go to your room after dinner. There will be no TV tonight." The child goes to his room, but later that night the father has to leave the house to go to a meeting. The mother then tells her son, "Come on in and watch TV. We won't tell Daddy."

> A child has been misbehaving in school and comes home with a lot of punish work. He does not start on it right away. His mother has been telling him time and time again to do the work. "If you are not finished by the time you're supposed to go to baseball practice, you're not going." Some time has passed, and he starts getting ready for practice. His mother asks him, "Didn't I tell you that you could not go if you didn't finish your work?" The child says, "I'm going, you can't stop me." Soon they are in a power struggle. The father hears the arguing and asks what's going on. The mother tells him what has happened and the boy gives his side of the story. Then the father says, "The team is depending on him. Now son, you go to practice and do your punish work when you come home." The boy leaves to play, with his parents arguing.

Parents can produce inconsistency by having different rules and expectations for their child, by undermining each other, and by not presenting a unified approach to the child. First, this produces confusion and unpredictability in the environment, which often increases the level of activity in overactive children. Second, the child is learning to play one parent against the other and to manipulate to get his or her way. When one parent disciplines or makes a comment and the other contradicts it, the first parent's authority is reduced. Consequently, the child views the second parent as the one who holds authority and will not listen to the other. Finally, this type of approach tends to identify one parent as the "bad guy" or the mean one and the other as the "good guy," the one who steps in and rescues the child or the one who has the more lenient rules.

Inconsistency also produces arguing between parents. When this happens, some children identify themselves as the cause of the conflict and may then view themselves as the root of all the conflicts their parents are having.

Inconsistency between parents or the primary people (babysitter, grandparents) dealing with the child on a daily basis leads to a very unpredictable management situation. The environment becomes unstructured and confusing when the primary people dealing with the child are approaching from different directions.

Therefore, it is extremely important for parents to be consistent as a unit. You should sit down with your spouse and try to set similar rules and expectations for your child's behavior. You do not always have to agree. But if you disagree with your partner it is best to support him or her in front of your child. Later, when your child is not around, discuss the situation and resolve it. For example, suppose your partner deprives your child of TV for a week because he did not want to go to bed when told. Although you may feel that the punishment is too severe, you should support him in front of the child and later resolve the difference of opinion. Perhaps you'll decide that the next time he gives you trouble about going to bed, he will have to go to bed earlier the next night. So when that behavior occurs again, a rule and consequence have been established, and you and your partner can present a unified front.

Although you should try to avoid this, punishment when changed should be changed by the individual who originally administered it, not the other parent. This can be done in two ways. First, the parent can simply tell the child, "I made a mistake and feel I was too hard on you," "I was angry and went overboard on your punishment," or whatever. "Therefore, I'm going to reduce it to one night," or whatever would seem more appropriate. A better way to reduce or change punishment would be to have a child "earn" his way out of the punishment. For example, "I told you that you were punished for a week, but after I've thought about it, we'll make it this way. Every night you go to bed when told without a hassle, that will take one night off your punishment." Or, "I have some jobs I want you to do around the house. For every one that is completed, you can take one day off your punishment."

DIFFERENT RESPONSES TO THE SAME BEHAVIOR

Depending on our mood, we often treat the same behavior in very different ways. For example, a child runs through the house today and you calmly explain that he should not run in the house because he may be hurt. Tomorrow he does the same thing and you scream and get upset. The next day he runs in the house and you send him to his room for ten minutes. The following day you are tired and ignore the behavior, and so forth. Different responses to the same behaviors also occur when we are disciplining our children. For example, one day your daughter might get a whipping for fighting with her sister. The next day she may be sent to her room. Another time the fighting might be overlooked.

When we respond to our children in this inconsistent fashion, we set up a situation similar to the following. Let's say today I see you and smile and shake your hand. Tomorrow I see you, smile, and punch you in the nose. The next time I see you, smile, and take your car away. Another day I smile and give you money. This goes on for several months. How are you going to respond to me when you see me? How are you going to feel?

First of all, you cannot predict my behavior. Although I am nice to you and doing good things for you at times, you do not know what to expect. Therefore, when you see me you will probably tighten up, be confused, and feel tense and somewhat insecure. You will probably try to place some physical distance between us and will not be able to become emotionally close to me or form a friendship. Children experiencing similar signals from their parents feel the same way. This unpredictable, inconsistent interaction is difficult for them to handle, and often their level of activity increases in response.

Although this cannot always be done, it is best to try to set up a specific consequence for each behavior. For example, it may be a standard rule in your house that whenever anybody runs they go to their room for five minutes. If you hit your sister, you lose ten minutes of TV time. If the toys are not picked up, you cannot play with them the next day. Setting up rules and consequences in this fashion will reduce inconsistency, make the environment more structured and predictable, and therefore, decrease the probability of problems.

CONSISTENCY IN THE ENVIRONMENT

Interpersonal consistency is very important in managing overactive children. However, routines also add to structure in the environment and reduce activity. For example, a child who has a set bedtime will give you less trouble when it is time to go to bed than a child who retires at different times. Homework will be less of a chore if it is done at the same time each day. Baths, feeding the pets, putting the garbage out, and so on will require less reminding if a routine is established. You do not have to make your home like a military operation, but you should try to structure it as much as you reasonably can. Try to establish routines to make the environment more predictable for the child.

Consistency may seem like a minor concept, but it adds a significant amount of structure to the environment. It serves as a foundation on which other behavior management techniques are built. A good rule to keep in mind when interacting with your child is: Do not say anything you can't or don't want to do, and do everything you say you are going to do. You have to follow through for any intervention to work. The structure and predictability provided by a consistent approach will often significantly reduce overactive behaviors.

SETTING RULES

Another major method by which structure and predictability are added to the environment is the way parents set and enforce rules, in other words, how we tell our children what we expect or what we want them to do. We usually have thousands of rules and regulations around the house. For example, "pick up your clothes, sit still while eating, stop being sassy, don't jump on the sofa." Parents are usually excellent in specifying what they want or in setting a rule.

NEGATIVE EFFECTS OF RANDOM DISCIPLINE

Parents set the rules well, but if the child breaks the rule or does not live up to the behavioral expectations, mistakes are made. If the child at grandmother's does not do what he is told, the parent then decides what is going to happen—whether the child gets hollered at, goes home, or gets a whipping or lecture. When the child comes home late, the parent decides if the child goes to her room, can't go out and play the next day, or gets her bike taken away for the week. We state the expectation beautifully, but we wait till the rule is broken and *then* we decide what the consequence will be. This can be termed *random discipline*. When we discipline or try to enforce rules and expectations in this fashion, several consequences make effective child management difficult.

Random Discipline Creates an
Unpredictable Environment

By being disciplined after the rule is broken, the child does not know what to expect. His or her environment lacks structure and predictability, and increased levels of activity become a greater possibility.

Random Discipline Does Not Make the
Child Feel Responsible

When random discipline is used the child does not feel in control of the consequences of his or her behavior and often feels that others are responsible for what has happened. For example, you try to get a child to stop aggravating his sister and tell him, "Stop doing that. Leave your sister alone. I've told you forty times to leave your sister alone. Now go to your room." Why is the child in his room? Because you have decided to send him there. Many children in similar situations have told me, "If I knew they were going to take my bike away for a week for riding on that street, I wouldn't have done that. But they didn't tell me what was going to happen. All they said was, 'Don't ride your bike on Judge Perez Drive.' "

In other words, children do not develop responsibility and tend to feel others determine what happens to them. They then tend to blame others for what has happened to them. "The teacher didn't tell us we should study that, that's why I failed the test." "Daddy hollered at me, that's why I broke my toy."

Random Discipline Creates Anger

If parents wait till children break the rule and then decide what will happen, children are likely to develop anger toward them because they feel their parents are responsible for the bad things (discipline) that have happened to them. When rules are enforced in this fashion, children are justified in being angry and feeling out of control of the consequences of their behavior.

To understand how children feel under these circumstances, let's take an example pertaining to work and paychecks. Say that you go to work and your boss tells you exactly what he expects of you. "Come to work every day. You have an hour for lunch. You work from 8:00 A.M. to 5:00 P.M.," and so forth. He spells out the rules and expectations very clearly. After you have been working for him for a few weeks, you miss a day of work and receive a paycheck that is $5 less than your usual one. The next week you miss a day and your check is $100 short. Another week you stay home a day and your boss deducts $35 from your check. After a couple of months of this, you go up to the boss and say, "What's going on? I miss work and you're taking out of my check all different amounts of money." The boss responds, "That's what I think you deserve for doing that. I needed you on the day I took out $100, but I didn't need you when I just deducted $5."

As the employee you would be angry and think your boss was unfair. You would also feel he is responsible for what is happening to you, and you would tend to blame him for your behavior. For example, a friend asks you, "Why didn't you buy that TV you said you were going to buy?" You would probably respond, "My boss took a lot of money from my paycheck, and now I can't buy it." You would make him responsible.

Such situations occur many times a day in most families. The parent decides what will happen to the child after he or she breaks a rule or does not behave as expected. A child will have a difficult time developing responsibility if disciplined in this manner. He may develop anger and resentment toward his parents, be confused, and have a difficult time knowing where he stands. In addition, she may have trouble becoming emotionally close to a parent who responds to her in this fashion.

Random Discipline Makes Parents
Feel Guilty

Also when parents discipline in this fashion, they tend to feel guilty for what they have done and try to undo it. This results in an inconsistent approach to the child. For example, you and your children are watching their favorite program on TV, and the kids are fighting and teasing each other. You have told them repeatedly to stop and behave, but they continue. You finally reach your breaking point and tell them, "I've told you 100 times to stop but you will not listen. Now go to your room, you can't watch TV." You start reading the newspaper. Then you start thinking; you feel mean, guilty, or upset for what you've done—"Maybe I was a little too hard on them. I've made them miss their favorite program." After some thinking, you really feel like a bad guy. You go to their rooms and ask them if they can be good, and in a few minutes they are back watching TV and you have eliminated your guilt feelings. However, nothing constructive has been accomplished, the environment has become inconsistent and structure has been lost.

CLEARLY DEFINED RULES AND CONSEQUENCES

In setting rules not only should we state the expectations, but, more important, we should state the consequences *before* the rule is broken. Both the rule and the consequences of the child's behavior must be clearly spelled out. When this is done, the environment becomes very predictable and structured. The child knows exactly where he or she stands and what will happen in response to certain behaviors.

Let's take the example pertaining to work and paychecks to see how it is done. We come to work and the boss states the rules or expectations. "Come to work every day. You have an hour for lunch. You work from 8:00 A.M. to 5:00 P.M.," and so forth. But this time he takes it a step further and also states the consequences. "The days you come to work and are here a full day you will be paid $35." Now each day you miss work, your weekly check is $35 short. At the end of two months you look at your check stubs; there is a $35 deduction for each day you missed. By having the expectations and consequences spelled out in this fashion, you cannot make your boss responsible for the deductions. There is only one person to blame—yourself. You are responsible for what has happened to you. Your friend asks you, "Why didn't you buy that TV you said you were going to buy?" Now you should respond, "Well, I decided not to go to work, so I didn't get a full paycheck. Now I don't have enough money to buy the TV." In setting up the rules and consequences in this fashion, your boss has made you accountable for your own behavior. You know exactly what is going to happen, and you can predict the consequences of your behavior.

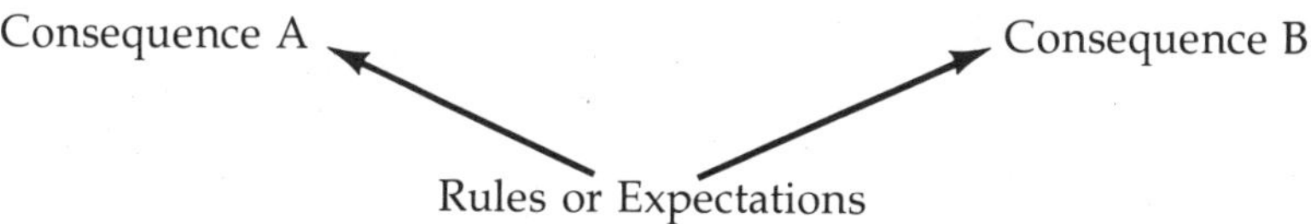

The above diagram indicates the way effective rules should be set. That is, you should tell your children, "Here is what I want you to do. This (Consequence A) will happen if you do it that way, and this (Consequence B) will happen if it is done the other way." Now the child will actually decide for him or her self what is going to happen.

A few examples of some everyday behaviors will illustrate the principle.

Running through the house: "I do not want you running through the house. You may get hurt or knock down your brother. Every time you run through the house, I am going to put a check on the piece of paper on your door. For every check you have by tonight, you will go to bed ten minutes earlier than the usual time."

Taking a bath: "I would like you to go take your bath. If you are in the bathtub by 6:30 P.M., washed, and out by 7:00 P.M., you can stay up thirty minutes past your bedtime. However, if that's not done, you will have to go to bed at the same time as you do every night."

Picking up toys: "You can go outside and play as soon as your toys are picked up. If they are not picked up you cannot go outside and play."

Sassiness: "I don't like you talking back to me and raising your voice. As long as you talk in a normal tone, you can go about your normal business. However, each time you are sassy, you will have to go in your room for fifteen minutes."

Putting things where they belong: "Your bike should be put in the backyard and not left in the front of the house. When it is not put where it is supposed to go, you will not be able to ride it the next day. If it is placed in the proper place, you can continue riding it."

Doing homework: "You mentioned to Daddy that you want to go to the basketball game Friday night. That's fine, but you know we have been having a lot of trouble getting you to do your homework. I'll tell you what we will do. If you come home three out of the four days this week and do your homework without a hassle, you can go to the game. However, if you give us trouble about the homework more than one time this week, you will not be able to go to the game."

Dinner time: "You are always getting up and moving around while we are eating. If you stay still and do not get up more than three times while we are eating, we will play that game you like to play. If you get up more than three times, we will not play the game."

Coming home on time: "You have been having some trouble coming home on time. You are supposed to be home by 5:00 P.M. to eat, but you are always late, and I know you are aware of the time. On the days that you come home on time, you will be able to have a snack at night. When you are late, I am going to come get you, and you will not be allowed to have a snack that night."

Fighting between siblings: "As soon as you walk in from school, the teasing and fighting starts and it doesn't seem to end. Starting today, if you can keep the fighting down and get along till after supper time, we will take a ride and get some ice cream after we eat. If you cut up, we don't go."

In these examples the parent is in control. That is, the adult specifies the expectations and consequences. However, the child decides what will happen. A map is drawn, and all you have to do is wait for your child to tell you what to do. You don't have to nag. The child, by his or her behavior, will tell you whether he wants to stay up past his bedtime, go to her room, go to the basketball game, and so on. Then all you have to do is be consistent and follow through with the consequence the child chooses.

One of the most important things to teach our children is that they are responsible for their own behavior—if good things happen it is because of them, and if bad things happen they are caused by them also. A lot of adults never learn responsibility for the consequences of their behavior. If children feel they are responsible for the consequences of their behavior, they can change situations. If things are bad they can make them better, and if they are happy with what is happening they can maintain it. However, if they feel that their parent is responsible, they are like puppets on a string and have to wait till others decide to make them feel good.

Therefore, in setting rules the parent should tell the child not only what is expected, but, more important, what is going to happen if he or she does one thing or another. The child then decides what the consequences will be. Consequences are the most important things in changing behavior.

Expectations and Consequences Should Be Stated One at a Time

Overactive children often have difficulty following a series of directions. Therefore, if several rules and consequences are given at once, there is a strong probability that some will not be followed. State rules and consequences one at a time. Also, be sure the child hears what you say. Overactive children are often distractible and may not hear what you have said. A good practice is to have the child repeat the rule and consequence after you have stated it. By doing this, you can see if the child understands or has heard the rule. At first, you may also have to remind him or her about it.

Expectations and Consequences Must Be Specific

How many times has something like this happened to you? Your child's room has been messed up for three weeks; it seems like everything he owns is on the floor. You tell him, "Go in your room and get all that stuff off the floor." About ten minutes later he comes out of his room and you ask, "Did you do what I said?" His response is "Yes." You go in the room and find all the junk that was on the floor now on the bed. What has happened? The child has taken you literally and has fulfilled your expectation 100 percent.

One morning I was getting ready to go to work and my wife was trying to get my oldest boy up to go to school, but he would not budge and continued sleeping. I passed his room and said something like, "You better be out of the bed by the time I'm finished shaving." When I finished I went to check on him, and sure enough he had done exactly what I told him. He had taken his pillow and blanket off his bed and was now sleeping on the floor.

Children often do *exactly* what you tell them. Therefore, in stating rules or behavioral expectations, you should be as specific as possible. "I want you to go in your room and put your toys where they belong and the dirty clothes in the bathroom." "Walk in the house. Any other means of getting from one place to another will result in your losing ten minutes of TV time."

Parents are also apt to encounter problems in management if the expectations or consequences are stated in too general terms. For example, "I want you to behave when we go to the shopping center" or "I want you to be good this afternoon." What does *behave* or *good* mean? It means different things to different people. Being good for an eight year old might mean hitting his sister only ten times instead of twenty-five times. Whereas the parent defines being good as not hitting his sister at all. Therefore, when the child and parent compare notes, they come up with different answers. The parent feels the child has misbehaved, but the child feels the opposite and believes he or she has been unfairly disciplined.

The same thing happens when you state consequences in general terms. "If you do that again, you are going to get it." "If you don't pick up your toys, you'll be punished." What does this mean to a child? Probably not very much.

In stating expectations or rules and consequences, you must be very specific and spell out exactly what you mean. You cannot assume that the child "knows." Both parent and child have to have the same idea of what is expected and what the consequences will be. It should not be a mystery or guessing game for the child. If it is, the child is apt to be confused and develop resentment for being disciplined.

GENERAL WAYS TO SET UP
EXPECTATIONS AND CONSEQUENCES

Expectations and consequences must be spelled out ahead of time to be most effective. The three general ways to accomplish this follow.

Natural Consequences

Some behaviors carry with them natural consequences, and these are often sufficient to produce change. If I beat my head on the floor, the natural consequence is that my head will hurt, and that may be enough to prevent me from continuing the behavior. If the only thing a child obtains by having a temper tantrum is a sore throat, upset stomach, or hurting head that behavior will quickly decrease. Natural consequences are often a good way to start to manage some problem behaviors.

Many children have eating problems, and mealtime for some families is a hassle. One way to begin to change picky eating or lack of eating is by natural consequences. A house rule may be that "dinner is served between 5:00 P.M. and 6:00 P.M. Those who eat can have a snack tonight. Those who do not will have nothing to eat tonight." Hunger is often a very powerful natural consequence to change behavior.

When I suggest this method to some parents, they say, "You want me to starve my child?" Most children's eating problems result from the way they are handled by the parents. Eating is a biological drive. You have to eat to live. It's not like doing homework, picking up toys, not being sassy, because you do not have to do these behaviors to survive. In addition, it has been shown that a person has to fast for several days before significant effects develop. Parents often teach faulty eating patterns. The picky eater has a specially prepared dinner. When a child does not eat dinner, he comes to the parent later and says, "Can I have some milk and cookies?" Although you want to say "no," you think, "He didn't eat, so at least he'll have something in his stomach before he goes to bed." Therefore, the child starts developing an unusual eating pattern that could probably have been prevented by using the natural consequence of hunger.

Bed-wetting is another behavior where natural consequences can easily be used. If you wet the bed, you have to change your clothes, make the bed, wash your clothes, or whatever duties the child is physically capable of performing. Therefore, if you wet the bed you are held accountable for the consequences of that behavior.

Children often "get sick" to avoid unpleasant situations, such as school, tests, or other obligations. Then when they get home, or when the other children are home to play, they recover very rapidly. Natural consequences can also be used here. "If you're sick, you'll have to go to the doctor"—most kids don't love that. Or the house rule could be that when people are sick they remain in their room, in bed, without play or TV time. Therefore, the positive consequences of not being sick far overweigh the negative natural consequences of being sick.

Parents who have trouble with children putting their dirty clothes in the proper place may state, "I only wash clothes that are in the dirty clothes basket. Those left in other places will not be washed." In this situation, the natural consequence of leaving your favorite T-shirt or jeans in your room is that it remains dirty, and you cannot wear it.

In all of the above situations, you must respond in a matter-of-fact manner and not get upset. Consistency and following through with what is said are also extremely important.

Grandma's Rule

This is a principle that most parents use frequently, and it can be stated very simply: you first do what I want you to do, then you can do what you want to do. Our grandmother or parents often said, "Eat your meat and potatoes and then you can have your dessert." This method of setting consequences can be used on the spur of the moment. However, it usually has to involve some activity that interests the child. For example, you are having a lot of difficulty getting a child ready for school and you know he enjoys watching TV before going to school. Using grandma's rule you would say, "The TV is not turned on until you're dressed and ready for school."

> "We will take a ride to get some ice cream as soon as all these toys are picked up."

"If you go play quietly for a few minutes, I'll play with you after I wash the dishes."

"You will get your snack as soon as you're dressed for bed."

"No one watches TV until all the homework is completed."

"We will play a game as soon as you take your bath."

"You cannot go outside and play until your room is clean."

In all of these examples you are setting expectations and consequences and giving the child a decision to make. As parents, all you do is carry out what the child tells you to do. In the last example, we are actually saying, "I would like you to clean your room. When you pick up your room, you can go outside. If it's not clean you stay inside."

Arbitrarily Set Consequences
When natural consequences or grandma's rule cannot be used, we identify consequences that are important to the child and set our rules or behavioral expectations according to these.

A child might be sassy. You know she does not like to stay in her room. Therefore, you might tell her, "I don't like you talking back to me and being sassy. Each time this happens you will have to go to your room for fifteen minutes."

Another child may not be bringing home his homework assignment and because of this may be doing poorly in school. You know that he loves to stay up past his bedtime. You may tell this fellow, "For every homework assignment you bring home and complete you can stay up five minutes past your bedtime."

Picking up toys or straightening up a room might produce a hassle in your family. If your child loves to play games you may tell her, "I am going to check your room at 7:00 P.M., and if it is clean and your toys are put away, we will play a game. On the nights it is not clean we will not play any games."

Another child loves to watch TV but has difficulty getting along with his brother and continually teases him. You might say, "Each time you tease your brother, you will lose ten minutes of TV time."

In these examples you identify a consequence that is important to the child and then set the behavioral expectations according to this.

It is not a natural consequence or something that follows an activity, but something that is individualized according to the child's interests. The consequence could be positive (reward) or negative (punishment).

chapter four

REWARDS OR POSITIVE CONSEQUENCES

Consequences are very important in managing and changing child behavior. The previous section discussed the most effective ways to use them to produce a structured, consistent, and predictable environment. Now we will examine the three general types of consequences that parents can use in managing their children.

Most parents usually rely on only one consequence to discipline overactive children—punishment. By *punishment* I mean negative attention, emphasis on bad behavior, anything from hollering at a child to whipping him. Many times a week I hear, "I've tried everything on this child, but nothing works!" The first question I ask is, "What have you tried?" The usual answers I get are "I've taken him off the baseball team, put him in his room, wouldn't let her play outside, made her write lines." What most parents are telling me is that they have used every form of *punishment* that they could dream up. Most parents are punishers. That is, they pay more attention to misbehavior than to appropriate behavior. If everything is going OK, we tend to not say anything, but let something go wrong and we are quick to notice it.

A child brings home a report card with ten As, ten Bs, three Cs, and one F. You spend a minute talking about the As, Bs, and Cs and an hour and a half on the F.

You tell a child to go clean the kitchen, and he goes in and does a wonderful job but leaves a glass on the counter and does not put the mop where it belongs. The child calls you to inspect the kitchen—what is the first thing you say? "Pick up that glass. Put the mop in the locker." Although 99 percent of the job has been completed perfectly, you comment only on the part that was done incorrectly.

A child is supposed to put her bike in the backyard and not leave it in front of the house. She puts it in the backyard ten days, and the eleventh day leaves it in the front. When do you think the child gets attention for this behavior? The day she did not put it away. Nobody says anything on the other days.

You tell your child, "I want you home at 5:00 P.M., no later. If you come home late, you will take your bath and go to bed." What happens if the child comes home late? You give her a lot of attention. That is, you holler at her, or give her a lecture. What happens if she comes home on time? Nothing. She just avoids negative attention.

The point is, we usually stress bad behavior. This may be because such disciplinary tactics were used on us, or this is how society operates, or whatever. Nevertheless, it happens.

Most professionals involved in managing overactive children or in providing parents with techniques to live with, interact with, and discipline their children more effectively stress a positive approach. That is, shift the emphasis from what the child does wrong to what he or she is doing right. In doing this, the parent pays more attention to good behavior and less to inappropriate actions or misbehavior.

A positive approach to your child's behavior can be accomplished by attending to everyday, normal behaviors and behaviors that are successful and appropriate. For example, noting the days the bike was put in the correct place, the clean areas of the kitchen, and the As, Bs, and Cs on the report card. This is particularly important for overactive children because much of their behavior requires correction (e.g., "don't touch that," "sit still," "quit teasing your sister"). Although you want to overlook some of the child's "bad" behaviors, I am *not* saying you should avoid correcting or pointing out the negative behaviors. Strive for a balance of attention to the child's positive and negative actions. If you dealt with your child three times today and all three focused on her mistakes, what she forgot to do, and so on, this would be worse than if you dealt with her one hundred times and fifty focused on her positive behaviors and fifty on her negative. Therefore, at the end of the day when you review your dealings with your child, strive for a balance. With the overactive child, you might want to overemphasize the positive direction a little.

This positive approach can also be accomplished by using the consequence of reward. When parents tell me, "I've tried everything," I usually say, "Have you tried rewarding him for doing good?" Often this is something that has never crossed their minds. Then, most parents have the wrong idea of what is meant by reward; they usually view it as a bribe. *Reward* can be defined simply as something that will serve as an incentive, anything that is important to the child. It is something that will increase the probability that the behavior will recur.

TYPES OF REWARDS

Rewards could be almost anything. Some general types follow.

Activity Rewards

These simply could be some activity that is of importance to the child—staying up past his bedtime, having a friend sleep over, playing a game with her mother, staying out later on Saturday, going to sleep at his grandmother's house, playing catch with her father, extra time to ride his bike, extra TV time, going to a dance or football game.

Foolish Rewards

Foolish rewards usually involve an activity that parents view as foolish or as work, an unlikely pleasure, but one the child views as a reward—washing the car, cutting the grass, using the vacuum cleaner, taking a shower, bringing a flower to the teacher, helping mother cook.

Material Rewards

These are usually concrete or material things that are of interest to the child—an extra dime for school, a toy, candy, a snack at night, a bag of potato chips, football cards, a record album, a basketball.

Things You Would Usually Buy

These rewards usually involve material things that parents would get for their child anyway. A child comes home and says, "I want a kite." More than likely you would buy her one, instead of doing this, you might use the kite as a reward.

Another child might say, "Joey has a pair of new tennis shoes. I wish I had some like his." You look at his shoes; they are old and he needs a new pair. However, this could be used as an incentive to change behavior.

Instead of just receiving them for no reason, these become rewards set up so the child can earn them. For example, the kite could be earned for not running in the house. The tennis shoes might be related to lack of sassiness.

Token Rewards

Token rewards have little value in themselves, but they represent something important or can be traded in for a desired object. For instance, money serves as a powerful token reward for adults. The kindergarten child who will behave or perform in school to get a star placed on his forehead or a happy face stamp on her hand is actually working for a token reward. These things represent approval, positive attention, and acceptance. Points or stars on a chart often serve as tokens that can be traded in for some desired object or activity.

Social Rewards

Social rewards are the most powerful rewards parents have, and they are carried around with us all the time. They do not cost a penny and can be simply defined as praise, recognition, and positive attention for good behavior. A majority of children will do a lot to get social rewards. They are not given often in some families, but frequently they are sufficient to change or maintain behavior. Social rewards could be verbal approval, telling the child he has done a good job, giving her a smile, a hug, or a kiss. They could be recognizing that he helped you set the table, giving attention to an everyday behavior (i.e., picking up clothes or brushing teeth), telling your child how pleased or proud you are of her, and offering various forms of praise.

Social reward, praise, positive attention, or nonverbal approval of good, appropriate behavior is a major part of the total approach to child behavior described in this book. It should be used with all of the rewards described above. That is, if a child earns an activity reward (e.g., staying up past her bedtime) for not being sassy, you should also praise the child for this behavior change.

Intrinsic Rewards

Intrinsic reward is self-reward, or behavior that is performed because it feels good. Patting yourself on the back for a job well done or engaging in a behavior because you enjoy it are types of intrinsic reward.

You have just finished reading a book. Your friend says, "What did you get out of that book? Did it tell you how to fix your car, build a house, or make spaghetti?" You reply, "I read it because I enjoyed it. It was fun to read."

You stop and help a boy whose car is broken down on the interstate—why? Probably because it makes you feel good to help someone in trouble.

Although I will emphasize material, social, and activity rewards, the purpose of these approaches is to get your child eventually to function on intrinsic rewards. That is, children should do things because they enjoy them or because it makes them feel good to engage in the behaviors.

QUESTIONS ABOUT REWARDS

When I start talking about reward several questions are usually asked by parents who do not agree with this philosophy. They bring us to a discussion of the purpose of reward.

Are you telling me to bribe my child to be good? The answer to this question is *no*. A bribe can be defined as paying someone to do something that is illegal, giving a person something for an inappropriate behavior. For example, you get a traffic ticket, and you pay somebody to fix it. I go to work every day and do not feel it is because of a bribe. You would probably think it was foolish if someone would say, "Your boss bribes you to go to work." You and I go to work because of consequences. The positive consequences (reward) of going to work are greater than those of staying home. Therefore, we show up at work every day. If parents are in control and set behavioral expectations and consequences, they are doing the same thing an employer does to get her employee to come to work. By using rewards parents can set up situations so that a child will want to behave in an appropriate fashion because the positive consequences of being good will far outweigh the consequences of not doing what is expected.

You're telling me to pay or reward my child for something he's supposed to do? Children learn what is right and wrong and what they are supposed to do. When they are born they do not know: "I'm supposed to be still. I should not talk back to my parents. I'm supposed to get along with my sister and not tease her." Therefore, if a child is not doing what he is supposed to do, we can assume that he has not learned to. Using positive consequences is one very effective way to teach a child what he should and should not do.

Won't my child learn to misbehave to get rewarded? With this statement parents are saying, "My child will become a con artist and will learn to manipulate me by bad conduct to get paid for being good." This will not happen if parents are in control and are setting the expectations and consequences. Manipulation will primarily occur if parents are inconsistent or if the child is in control. For example, a parent tells a child twenty times, "Go pick up your toys," but she does not respond. Then the parent says, "If you pick up your toys, I'll give you a dollar." Or a child misbehaves and then says, "What are you going to give me if I'm good?"

Parents need to be very consistent and in control to prevent manipulative behavior from developing. You must follow through with what is said, and you need to set the rules and consequences.

Am I going to have to reward this child the rest of her life for being good? The answer to this question is *yes* and *no*. Parents should continue using social reward for good behavior throughout the child's life. This type of reward should always be present in family interaction. However, material and activity rewards should be phased out as soon as possible, because the goal of this system is to get the child functioning on intrinsic reward.

The primary purpose of reward is to get a child to want to do what is asked or expected. Reward often changes the child's motivation. It will change a behavior that the child views as undesirable into something he wants to do. Once this is accomplished, we have half the ball game won. Let's take an example. Suppose a child views getting dressed for school as an undesirable behavior, and you have difficulty getting her dressed and ready each morning. Some common approaches to the situation are: hollering at the child, dressing her, criticizing, punishing.

A positive approach using reward might follow this procedure. First an incentive or reward would be identified. Let's say the child loves potato chips (but you could use anything that would be important to her). You tell her, "When I wake you up for school, I am going to set the timer on the stove for fifteen minutes. If you are dressed when the bell rings, we will stop on the way to school and get a bag of potato chips. If you are not dressed, we do not get the chips." The aim of this reward is *not* to continue giving the child a bag of potato chips until she is a junior in college for getting dressed in the morning. The purpose is to change an undesirable action into a behavior that the child wants to do.

During the time she is getting dressed for school, you are praising her and giving her new behavior a lot of attention. You will see that the first and second week the child cannot wait to get to the store to get the potato chips. By about the third or fourth week the chips will become less important; she may not ask to get them in the morning, but she is still getting dressed for school. The purpose of the reward or incentive is to make her want to do something that she previously thought was undesirable. Once you can get her to do it, you are halfway to changing the behavior. When she is doing what you want, all you have to do is associate verbal approval and praise with the new behavior. Eventually, the child will engage in the behavior because it is more enjoyable and pleasurable (intrinsic reward) to get dressed on time than to fool around and get hollered at, punished, and be late.

Therefore, start with material or activity rewards to motivate the child to engage in the new behavior. Once the child changes behavior, use social reward, and eventually the material reward can be phased out. Finally, intrinsic rewards will take over.

The following is a somewhat silly example, but it will stress these points. Let's say I ask you, "Would you please go in your yard and count the blades of grass for me? Separate the different types of grass, the light green ones from the dark green ones. I'll be back tomorrow to get the results, and I'll give you $5." What would you think? You would not want to do what I asked, probably think I was nuts for asking you to do that, and you would not count the grass. That behavior is undesirable, something you do not want to do (like doing homework, picking up clothes, not being sassy, or any other problem behavior that you see in your child). Now, let me rephrase my request. "Would you please go in your yard and count the blades of grass for me? Separate the different types of grass, the light green ones from the dark green ones. I'll be back tomorrow to get the results and I'll give you $1,500." Now, you would probably stay by your house to count the grass to get the $1,500. What have I done? By using a reward, I have increased your desire to engage in a behavior you thought I was crazy to ask you to do. I have changed an undesirable behavior into something you want to do. Let me stretch a point in this silly example to emphasize the process that occurs when reward is used effectively.

Let's assume that I am an important person to you, like your mother or father, and I can get you to count grass everyday. When you do what I ask you to do, I use social reward and say, "You're doing a beautiful job. I'm proud of you and never knew you could do this so well. I never saw people count grass so fast, etc." What is going to happen eventually is that my praise will gain importance and the material reward will not be as important. Soon you will be counting grass to receive social reward. The next step would have intrinsic reward taking over. You would engage in the behavior because you enjoyed it and derived pleasure from it.

Although this is an extreme example, much of your behavior is already based on intrinsic reward. For example, people start working to eat and have money. However, many have enough money; they do not have to work or can retire, but instead they continue working for the pleasure. Some people get involved in coaching Little League baseball or engage in other behaviors that require a lot of effort just for enjoyment.

Positive consequences or rewards are extremely important in dealing with overactive children; they should be used as the main disciplinary tactic or method of control, because some misbehaviors may be beyond the child's control. Let's say you have a child who fidgets or who's overtalkative during mealtime. Suppose punishment is used to deal with this behavior, and the child cannot change his actions. This would be like punishing him for breathing. However, if you use reward to deal with this behavior, you will be able to determine if it can be controlled. If the child cannot change his actions, the discipline will be less frustrating and less likely to produce additional problems. For example, the child who gives problems during mealtime and loves to play ball with his father may be told, "I'm going to give you warnings during mealtime whenever you get up or squirm (or whatever the child is doing that is a problem). If you get three or less warnings, you will be able to go outside and play ball with your father. If you get more than three warnings, you will not be able to go outside and play ball." If you know the reward is important to the child and this procedure is used for several days, you will be able to determine if he can or cannot control the target behavior.

MAKING REWARD EFFECTIVE

Reward is a very powerful consequence and can be used to deal with overactive behavior. However, several things must be kept in mind for reward to work effectively.

Individualize Reward

A consequence that is rewarding for one child may not produce the same effect for another. When trying to identify a reward for a particular child, you have to look closely at that child's needs, interests, and habits. Some kids will work like crazy to earn 10¢, other children would not move a finger for a million dollars. Therefore, if you are using extra TV time for your daughter and it is working fine, do not automatically assume it will work for your son.

A statement I hear frequently is, "Nothing interests my child. I don't know what I can use as a reward." I have not met a child for whom a reward could not be identified. For some children a reward is easily found, but for others more detailed investigation is necessary. I usually tell the parents to listen to their children very carefully, observe their play, and ask the child what is important to him or what she would like to work toward. All children can be motivated by incentives, although for some they are more difficult to identify.

Always Use Social Reward

Regardless of the type of incentive used, social reward should *always* be paired with the behavior. The main purpose of material or activity reward is to motivate the child to want to behave in a certain fashion. Eventually, intrinsic reward should take over, but praise must be used for this to occur.

Don't Put the Cart Before the Horse

Parents often make the mistake of rewarding the child *before* the behavior. For example, "I'm going to buy you this bike, and because I've done this I want you to be good at school." On entering a supermarket you tell a child who usually misbehaves in stores, "I'm going to buy you this candy. Now, I want you to listen to me and be good."

What usually happens if you pay someone to paint your house before the job is complete? It usually is done halfway or is not completed to your satisfaction. The same thing happens when you give a child a reward and then expect her to behave in a certain fashion. Reward should be based on behavior and should always *follow* the expected action to be effective. If it comes before the desired behavior, you cannot expect it to work.

Be Sure to Give Rewards Earned

PARENT: I've used that reward system you told me to use. It worked fine for a few days, but now nothing's happening.

PSYCHOLOGIST: Tell me about it. What exactly did you use for reward and how did you set it up?

PARENT: Well, we were going to work on his sassiness. We used staying up past his bedtime as the reward. If he was not sassy until his bedtime, he would be able to delay his bedtime by thirty minutes. It worked fine for about five days, but now he's just as sassy as before.

PSYCHOLOGIST: What exactly happened? Did he earn the reward?

PARENT: He did fine the first five days. No sassiness and he earned the thirty minutes, but he gave us so much trouble about getting dressed for bed or teasing his sister, we didn't let him stay up.

Often children earn rewards for one behavior, but get them taken away for doing something else. This is one sure way to destroy the effectiveness of a reward system. Rewards earned *must* be received. How would you feel if I told you, "Please clean this chair and I'll give you $25. Then clean this one and I'll give you another $25." You clean the first one and I give you $25. Then you say, "I don't feel like cleaning the other chair." Now I tell you, "Give me back the $25 you earned because you wouldn't clean the second chair." You would be angry, and if I took the money away it would be difficult for me to motivate you for the same behavior again. The same thing will happen if a child earns a reward, but the parent does not see that the child receives it. For example, a child earns a breakfast at McDonald's for being still while eating dinner, but her parent never takes her or keeps delaying the reward.

Administer Reward Immediately

If a child does something this minute, ideally he or she should be rewarded right now—not next week or next month. The effectiveness of a reward is, in part, based on how close it comes to the behavior you are trying to increase or control. How well a reward works is *not* based on quantity or expensiveness but immediacy. Let's take an example of a six year old who has trouble getting dressed for school, but one costs 25¢ and one costs $450. The motorcycles. One morning you could say, "I'm going to set the timer on the stove and if you're dressed by the time the bell rings, we'll stop and get a bag of potato chips on the way to school." The next morning you could tell him, "If you get dressed for school on time, we'll stop at the Honda place and get the motorcycle you've been wanting." Now, let's say both rewards work, and he gets dressed for school, but one costs 25¢ and one costs $450. The motorcycle is not going to change the behavior permanently any more than the bag of potato chips. School performance or behavior is better rewarded on a daily or weekly basis than after each report card or grading period.

It is not always possible to reward a child for her behavior immediately. Therefore, social or token rewards should frequently be used to provide immediate reinforcement for desirable behavior.

Reward Improvement

Often a reward system does not work because parents expect too much change too rapidly and they do not reward improvement. Many times parents say to me, "My child won't listen." We then set up a reward system to work on that behavior. Two weeks later the parents return and say, "He's still not listening." This may be a fact if you look at the overall behavior, but in changing behavior you have to break it down into steps and look for gradual improvement. For example, a child may not have been listening thirty times a day before you started the reward, and after two weeks the not-listening behavior is down to fifteen times a day. In terms of overall behavior he is still not listening, but he has improved his behavior by 50 percent.

Therefore, in using reward, the behavior or goals have to be broken down into small goals. You cannot attempt to change a behavior overnight. You have to look at where the child is now and where you want to go. A child who is not listening thirty times a day should be rewarded if she can decrease that rate to twenty times a day the first week. After that, the amount of improvement necessary to receive the reward can be increased each week. For example, the second week reward would be received for fifteen times a day, the third week ten times a day, and so on. Eventually, the child would be rewarded for listening all but three or five times a week. Usually, it is best to allow some room for error and not expect 100 percent improvement.

Change Reward as Necessary

The purpose of using reward is to change behavior, and in most cases interests and attitudes are also modified. Therefore, a reward that may initially be important to a child might lose its effectiveness with time and use. Suppose you enjoy steak dinners. I could probably motivate you by saying, "If you help me, I'll take you out to the restaurant of your choice for a steak dinner." However, if you have eaten steak every day for a week, I would not be able to motivate you or change your behavior with the same reward, because you would be tired of it.

Children respond in the same manner and either become tired of or lose interest in the same reward. If a reward has worked beautifully in the beginning but is no longer effective, it must be changed.

In addition, when first trying a reward, you should use it consistently for a period of time (usually a week or so) before you try another because it is not working. Often parents do identify a reward that is important to a child, but because it does not work the first, second, or third time it is used, they try another one. Rewards need to be varied, but not too fast.

Make Reward Attainable

When a reward system is first started, it should not be too complex or too hard. The goal should not require a great deal of change, and it should be set up so the child succeeds and receives the reward. You have to lock the child into the system. If you make it too hard at first and the child is not able to attain the behavioral goal and incentive, the whole system will probably fail.

Let's take an example of a child who is sassy. You find that the undesirable action occurs an average of ten times a day. So you set up a positive system to decrease the behavior. You tell the child, "We are going to put a check on this calendar each time you are sassy. If you only have two checks when it is time to go to bed, you can stay up thirty minutes past your bedtime." When it is time for bed, you and the child look at the calendar and find he has five checks, so he does not receive the reward. In this instance, the total system is likely to fail because the expectations were set too high. This child has actually improved his behavior by 50 percent and, in a sense, was punished for doing this. Pretty soon the child will become disgusted with the system.

A good rule to follow is to expect about 40 percent change at first. Therefore, in the above example, the child should have received a reward if he eliminated four sassy behaviors in a day and received six checks.

Often reward systems are made too complex or hard, that is, too much work or change is required for the child to receive the reward. For example, a child may have to

1. Get out of bed when called in the morning
2. Eat all his breakfast
3. Put his clothes up when he comes home from school
4. Do his homework
5. Come in on time from playing
6. Not fight with his brother

7. Pick up his toys
8. Take his bath when told

If he does all of this, the reward is having a story read to him at bedtime. In this example, the child will probably think, "The heck with this—it's not worth it."

Use Behavior to Be Changed as a Reward

Let's say a child is scared of the dark or going into a room by herself and must be accompanied by a parent. Your goal is to eliminate the dependent behavior, but this can also serve as the reward. She will not leave the den to go to her room to get a toy without someone with her. Initially you might tell her to "take one step out of the den and then I'll come with you." After she is successfully doing this, she would then be told to "Take two steps out of the den and then I'll come with you." This would gradually be increased before you accompany her the rest of the way.

This procedure was also used with a problem eater who would only eat french fries and bread for dinner. Although we were trying to increase the variety of food this child would eat, we used the french fries and bread as the reward. At first the parent would place half a spoon of rice or any other food on the plate and the child was required to taste it before he could have the french fries and bread. As the child increased the variety of foods he would taste, he found some that he liked (e.g., corn), and the portions of these were increased. It was then easy to have him eat this before he was rewarded with the french fries and bread. As the portions and variety of foods increased, he ate less and less of the reward and this unusual eating pattern diminished.

Some small children cannot play independently and require their parent, usually their mother, to amuse them continually. The parent might have the child play independently, sometimes in another room, for a few minutes and then play a game with her or read her a story. The time period is gradually increased so that she is required to show more independent play before receiving the reward.

This reward system can be very effectively used in a variety of situations. The procedure is to set up two behaviors that cannot exist at the same time. One behavior is the one that is to be increased and the other is used as the reward. For example, a child cannot be independent and dependent at the same time. By functioning on his own, he is rewarded with assistance. The amount of independent behavior to achieve the reward (depending) is increased and the behavior to be changed, or the reward, is decreased.

chapter five
PUNISHMENT OR NEGATIVE CONSEQUENCES

Most parents tend to pay more attention to their child's mistakes, failures, and misbehaviors than to their successes, achievements, and adaptive actions. By punishment, I mean any negative attention from hollering to whipping a child. For example, a child is supposed to make his bed or do some other chore every day. He does the chore six days, but forgets on the seventh day. The day he usually gets attention for his behavior is the day he does not do what you ask, while on the other days you usually do not say anything about his behavior. Another example would be a child who frequently runs through the house. Every time she runs she gets attention from her parents, but she gets little, if any, comments when she walks.

By responding to our children in this fashion, we set up a situation where the only thing the child receives for being good is not being punished or criticized. This type of parental response also results in children feeling that it is useless to do nice things because they are never good enough or no one pays attention to them. Children, like adults, avoid things that are negative. Therefore, if sitting down to do homework is a negative situation (it arouses a lot of punishment or hollering), the child tries to avoid homework and you have trouble getting her to do it. In addition, for some personality types, punishment actually makes matters worse.

Punishment should *not* be used as the main method of managing overactive children. The most effective way to use punishment is to combine it with other consequences. Rewarding and ignoring should be used about 60 percent to 70 percent of the time, with punishment being utilized 30 percent to 40 percent of the time.

NEGATIVE RESULTS OF PUNISHMENT

When punishment is used as a main method of control, some problems are apt to develop.

Overactive Children May Not Be Able
to Prevent Some Behaviors

Some behaviors (e.g., distractibility, short attention span, fidgetiness) in overactive children may be beyond their control. If punishment is used to change these behaviors, you may be punishing the child for something he or she cannot prevent. Therefore, this form of discipline as the main method of control may result in frustration, be detrimental to healthy personality development, or cause some of the problems described below.

Children Come to Behave out of Fear

If I came up to you and said, "I can get your child to do whatever you'd like him to do. I can do this in two ways. One way is out of fear of what's going to happen. The other way is because he's learning new behaviors or because he feels he's accomplishing something." Which method would you pick? Most people would pick the latter. However, most parents use the former.

Most forms of punishment are based on fear. "If you don't bring your grades up, you won't be able to play baseball this summer." "If you don't stop teasing your little sister, you are going to get a whipping." "You won't be able to go out and play tomorrow if you don't come home on time." Fear is not an emotion most parents would want to develop excessively in their children. When punishment is used as the main method of control, however, fear is repeatedly triggered.

Anger, Aggression, and Rebellion Often Develop

Using punishment as the main method of control will often produce anger and resentment toward the parents. This is especially true if the discipline is decided on and administered after the misbehavior, that is, if random discipline is used. Children that are primarily disciplined in this fashion often feel unjustly treated and develop considerable hostility toward their parents. Sometimes these feelings are expressed directly (e.g., "I hate you," "My father's mean"), but more often this anger is expressed through a variety of passive-aggressive behaviors, such as opposition, resistance, stubbornness, defiance, and rebellion. In addition, this anger may be displaced to other situations, and fighting with or anger toward siblings, peers, or other authority figures may be seen.

Emotional Distance Is Created
Between Parent and Child

Let's say you have a boss who controls you by fear (e.g., if you're not on time, you will be fired). He pays more attention to your mistakes than to your accomplishments. Whenever he comes around, you know he's going to criticize your work, and often you feel he unjustly disciplines and reprimands you. Would you feel close to this person, or would he become your friend? Would you feel secure and comfortable when he is around? No, you would probably not want to have anything to do with this individual and certainly would not want to visit socially with him or take him on a fishing trip with you.

When punishment is primarily used to discipline, children will often feel the same way about their parents. You do not feel close to people you are afraid of or who you feel give you more negative attention than positive recognition. Therefore, punishment fosters a significant amount of emotional distance between child and parent. This may ultimately result in a lack of verbal interaction (only talking to the parent when necessary) or withdrawal (spending more time alone in her room, minimizing contact with the family). Generally, a close emotional relationship in the family will fail to develop.

Escape or Avoidance Behaviors Develop

We all tend to avoid situations that produce negative attention. What would you do if every time you cooked gravy it turned out bad and you received a lot of criticism and negative attention? You would avoid it. Suppose every time you went to a friend's house she told you everything you were doing wrong and spent three hours talking about your failures and ten minutes on your accomplishments. How often would you want to go to her house?

Children often show the same feelings and behaviors when punishment is used as the main method of discipline. When fear and negative attention are used in discipline, avoidance and escape behaviors develop to avoid punishment. If every time a child cuts the grass all of his mistakes are pointed out, he'll learn to avoid grass cutting. When a child sits down to do her homework, if there is a lot of hollering or negative remarks, she will not want to do homework.

Lying, manipulating, running away from home, are avoidance behaviors learned by children who experience these situations. You hear a lamp fall off the table and break. Your youngest child is in the back room, and this is where the lamp was broken. You go into the room and say, "What happened? Did you break that lamp?" The child knows that if he says yes or admits to the behavior he'll get a great deal of negative attention. Therefore, he says, "I was watching TV and a band of gypsies came through the house and knocked over the lamp, and I don't know where they went after that. That's how it was broken."

Punishment Does Not Work
With Some Personality Types

Just as reward has to be individualized, so does punishment. For some personality types, punishment is sufficient to control behavior, but for others punishment does not work at all or only works for short periods of time.

Let's take an example of two children, Alan and Jason, sitting on the front porch while it is raining. Both want to go run in the rain and splash in the puddles. Jason is about to and is thinking, "If I run in the rain, I might be punished. I might get caught, and they might stop me from watching TV tonight, playing with my friends tomorrow, going to sleep at Preston's house Saturday, and so on." On the other hand, Alan is thinking, "I could really have fun running in the rain. I could try to run between the drops, splash in that big puddle, slide on the grass." These two children are getting ready to engage in the same behavior, but their motivations are different. For Jason, whether or not he runs in the rain depends on what negative consequences will happen to him. However, Alan's behavior is motivated by pleasure, that is what is in it for him. Jason can be controlled by punishment, but the pleasure-oriented Alan cannot. Reward has to be used to effectively deal with this child. In other words, we have to make it more pleasurable not to run in the rain than to do so.

It has been estimated that 30 percent to 40 percent of the children in the United States have Alan's personality type. Many overactive children seem to show this personality characteristic. Other consequences (reward and ignoring) have to be used to discipline these children.

Some Personality Types Develop
Personality or Emotional Problems

All children are different, and their responses to punishment are varied. Some children comply, others become angry or rebel, still others may withdraw, bottle up emotions, become nervous, feel guilty or fearful, have a negative self-image, or develop other emotional or personality problems. Because of the nature of their behaviors, overactive children receive a significant amount of negative attention.

One of the primary types of punishment used on children involves verbal negative attention. When used frequently, this interferes with healthy personality development and usually is a very ineffective method of discipline.

Hollering and screaming only create an emotional distance between parent and child and get both upset. Criticism and name calling only make the child feel bad about himself or herself. Controlling children by guilt (e.g., "I cook, take care of you, wash your clothes. Why aren't you good in school?" Or "I bought you that bike and took you out to eat and you still won't listen") or fear (e.g., "If you don't straighten up, I'll put you in a home." "If you and your sister don't stop fighting, I'm going to leave and let you take care of yourselves") develops unhealthy emotions.

Model Behaviors Develop Until . . .
Many times each month I hear, "My child didn't give me any problems until recently. He was a model child, but now he won't listen, does just the opposite of what I tell him, and generally I have a hard time controlling him. When he was little he did exactly what we told him and almost never objected to what we said. It's a different story now."

Where punishment is the main method of discipline, children with certain personalities often develop model behaviors when young. It often seems that these kids are "too good." However, somewhere between eleven and fourteen years of age all hell breaks loose. The anger that has been developing for years suddenly is seen and is primarily expressed through passive-aggressive attitudes. This type of personality often fools parents, but it doesn't last.

Effectiveness Is Lost When Many Behaviors
Receive the Same Punishment
Parents often overuse a certain type of punishment. A child may have to go to her room for being sassy, hitting her brother, not picking up her toys, coming home late, or whatever. Another child may receive a whipping for not being good at school, talking back to his mother, fighting, running in the house. Hollering is probably the most overused punishment. When you use one form of punishment for many different behaviors, the negative consequence is no longer important to the child, and it loses its effectiveness as a motivator.

It would be best to determine certain punishment for specific behaviors. That is, a child is sent to his room for being sassy or having temper tantrums and nothing else. Loss of TV time could be reserved for teasing her brother, and so forth.

Parents Serve as Models for Children's Behavior
Children learn behaviors by observing other people. This is called the *modeling theory of learning* and is the reason for not showing certain TV programs during family viewing hours. Children

exposed to certain behaviors will imitate them and may incorporate them into their patterns of dealing with conflicts, solving problems, and interacting with others.

Whether a child models a certain way of responding depends on two general factors: first, how similar the model is to the child, and second, how important or significant the model is in the child's eyes. Parents are the most significant people in their children's early lives, thus serving as very powerful models from which behavior is learned. Therefore, your children can learn many behavior patterns just by observing how you deal with situations, conflicts, and problems. Many times I hear a parent say, "He acts just like his father when he gets mad." "I get nervous very easily and so does my daughter." "My son's fears are similar to mine." The next thing that is said is, "He must have inherited that way of acting." For the most part, however, children are not born with these behaviors. They learn them. If a child sees his father throwing things when he is mad or dealing with conflicts by screaming, it is highly probable that this child will adopt these responses to similar situations. If a mother is fearful of storms, her child may also show this fear. To make this point with an extreme example, it has been found that a large percentage of parents who physically abuse their children were abused themselves as children.

Therefore, if you and your spouse deal with conflicts by arguing and screaming at each other, your child may be learning to deal with his or her siblings or peers in a similar fashion. This brings us to an important point regarding physical punishment (e.g., spanking or threats involving control by aggression or force). If I get a child in my office whose primary problem involves fighting, hitting other children, loss of temper, or trying to control others by physical means, the first questions I ask the parents are, "How is he disciplined? If he doesn't want to do something, how can you get him to do it?" The usual answers I get are: "I give him a whipping." "I tell him if he doesn't behave or do what I want, I'll give him a spanking." "I go get the belt." In these situations the child is being controlled by physical means or threats of aggression. Therefore, he is learning that if people do not do what you want, be aggressive, threaten them with force. So, when a child cuts in front of him in line at school, he shoves or hits him. If a child takes his pencil and will not give it back, a fight might start. The child's primary method of problem solving involves physical threats of aggression because he has modeled the significant people in his life, his parents.

Parents serve as significant models for children, and if a child lives with hostility, he learns to fight. If she lives with criticism, she learns to condemn, and so forth. If punishment is used as the main disciplinary tactic, your child may be adopting these methods to control others—peers, authority, siblings, and eventually his or her own children.

Punishment Changes Behavior Only Temporarily

Some people disagree on this point, but many experiments have proven that punishment does not result in a permanent or long-term change in a behavior pattern. The effects of punishment are only temporary, and after a period of time the punished behavior reappears. This is why some children show "good" behavior or a period of control after punishment that only lasts for a few days or a couple of minutes.

Let's say I tell you, "I'm going to drop by your house in ten minutes to have a cup of coffee." Your house is a mess, and you want it to look nice when I come over. So, you hurry up and try to make the house presentable. Things are stuffed in the closet, thrown behind the sofa, put under chairs, and so forth. Now, the house looks OK, but have you really changed anything? No, you have just rearranged things, and eventually you will have to go back and put everything in its proper place. This is how punishment often works. It only changes behavior on the surface, like sweeping dirt under the carpet.

When reward is used, the behavior is not changed as fast, but the improvement will be long lasting. To take the example above, reward would have the same effect as putting a few things where they belong. Although the house would not look as clean, it would be permanently changed, because you would not have to go back and put things away. They would be in their proper places, and if this procedure were gradually used the house would be clean.

When punishment is used as the main method of control, you can only expect the behavior to be modified for short periods of time. After a while, it will reappear and have to be dealt with again. The best way to use punishment is to sandwich it with reward.

Punishment Sometimes Maintains Misbehaviors

A phrase often overused in analyzing child behavior is, "He's doing that to get attention." While getting attention is frequently used inaccurately to explain certain behavior in children, this statement is sometimes true. That is, some kids often misbehave to get negative attention because this is better than nothing at all.

In other situations, children behave in certain ways to get a reaction from their parents. Whining, complaining, or being stubborn are often employed by children to make a parent nervous, upset, or frustrated and gain their own way. For example, your child says, "Can I go outside and play?" You say "No." Then the child starts complaining, whining, hitting his sister. After a few minutes of this, you are getting agitated and eventually you say, "Go outside and play. I'll call you when it's time to eat."

Children often behave in certain ways for attention as a method of expressing their anger or as a way to get back at their parents. For example, you tell your child, "Go to your room, you're punished." Now she's angry, she doesn't want to go to her room. What can she do? She cannot punch you in the nose, so she starts mumbling under her breath, saying things like, "You're mean. You like my brother better than me. I hate you and would rather live at Linda's house." Now you say, "What are you saying? Speak up. If I hear that again, you'll stay in your room longer." What has happened? You have given the behavior a great deal of attention, which is often sufficient to maintain it.

In the situation above, another problem also develops. You wind up punishing the child because of her reaction to the punishment, then punish her again because of her misbehavior, and so forth. Now, she has to stay in her room for four hours instead of fifteen minutes, and both you and she have forgotten what she was sent to her room for in the first place. The punishment snowballs, and the reason for the initial discipline is lost.

Misbehaving or behaving to get attention is usually not consciously planned by the child, but is often done unconsciously. One method of dealing with this type of behavior is ignoring (see Chapter 6).

Parents Feel Guilty and Unfair

This is especially true if punishment is administered in a random fashion, not spelled out ahead of time.

> A brother and sister are sitting in the room watching TV and they are constantly fighting. The mother has calmly told them ten times to quiet down and stop arguing, but this does not keep them from misbehaving. Finally, she starts screaming and eventually sends both of them to their rooms for the night. Now they will miss the Charlie Brown special coming on next. The mother, sitting in the quiet of the back room, starts thinking, "Maybe I was too hard on them. I shouldn't have done all that hollering, they were so good all day. They've been talking about the Charlie Brown special all afternoon and now I've made them miss it." Guilt starts to develop; the parent feels responsible for what has happened to the children. Next, she must undo what has happened to feel better. "Come on out of your room, you can watch TV if you are good."

Administering and reacting to punishment in this fashion results in a very inconsistent approach to child management, certain to result in ineffective discipline and continued misbehavior.

Punishment Often Does Not Offset the Reward Gained by the Misbehavior

> Your child comes up to you and says, "I'm hungry, can I have something to eat?" You say "No, we are going to eat in twenty minutes. If you eat something now, you'll ruin your appetite." You now have to leave the kitchen, and the child grabs a bag of cookies and goes into the back room and starts eating them. About fifteen minutes and twenty cookies later, you catch him with the goods and punish him for not listening and being sneaky. However, the behavior for which the child has been punished produced a great deal of reward, which the punishment will not offset.

> You have told your daughter to "come home when it's 5:00." She and her friends have spent from 3:30 to 5:00 building a jump to go over with their bikes. She knows it's time to come home, but she stays another half hour and makes forty jumps with her bike. She now shows up late and is punished.

One problem with punishment is that in some situations the behavior that is punished has received, or is receiving, reward. Therefore, if punishment is the main method of discipline, it will probably not counter the pleasure received for the misbehavior. This is one reason why punishment works more effectively when sandwiched with reward. Reward for appropriate behavior would produce better results than punishment for not listening.

TYPES OF PUNISHMENT

The types of punishment used by most parents can be grouped into five general areas. Some are effective; others should be used sparingly or avoided.

Response Cost

This is a very effective form of punishment and can be seen as a system where the child is fined or loses privileges or desired activities for misbehavior. "When you do something bad, it is going to cost you something." This is used frequently in our daily lives. For example, if you receive a speeding ticket, you have to pay a fine; when your income tax is late you are assessed a penalty.

A good example of a response cost system is allowance based on daily chores. Let's say a child has to feed the pet each day and put out the garbage five times a week. For these chores he gets an allowance of $3 each week. He has to perform twelve tasks each week to earn his full allowance (25¢ a task). A record on a calendar or a chart of his performance would be kept. Each time he performed the required duty without being told, 25¢ toward his weekly allowance would be earned. However, if the task was not performed by a certain time and the child had to be reminded, it would cost him 25¢. Therefore, it would be totally up to the child if he earns nothing or his full allowance each week.

I have used loss of money as punishment because a response cost system can easily be described in this fashion. However, the fine or thing lost could be any privilege or activity.

> For a child who loves to watch TV but is very sassy you could set up a response cost system using loss of TV time as the fine for sassiness. A chart could be constructed to keep a tally of the number of times a day sassiness appears. The child would then be told, "Each time you are sassy [the parents would specifically explain what they meant by sassiness] I am going to put a mark on this chart. At the end of the day, we will get a total, and for each mark you have you will lose ten minutes of TV time. Therefore, how much TV you watch each night is up to you and how well you can control your sassiness."

> Another example would be a child who has trouble coming home on time. She is always late or never comes inside when she is called. With a response cost system the child would be told, "For every minute that you are late or do not come inside when I call you, you

> will lose that much play time [TV time, reading time at night, or something similar could be used] the next day." So, if she is supposed to come home each day at 5:00 but she comes thirty minutes late today, tomorrow she would be required to come home at 4:30.

Any type of activity, privilege, or thing that is important to the child can be used as the "fine" in a response cost system of punishment. However, several points must be kept in mind. First, you have to define clearly the behaviors that will be fined and exactly what they will cost the child. Second, it has been proven that this type of system works best when positive consequences or rewards are also being used. Third, do *not* set up a system where the child will owe you or the loss will become unrealistic. If a child gets $3 a week allowance and the parent says, "Each time you're sassy you will lose 25¢ of your allowance, the child may have a minus allowance at the end of the week and owe the parent $5. Or a parent may tell a child, "Each time you hit your brother, you will have to go to bed ten minutes early." If this child hits his brother enough, he may wind up going to bed when he comes home from school! This type of response cost is sure to fail. Finally, the fines have to be consistently given when the misbehavior occurs.

Time Out

Time out also is an effective form of punishment and is used frequently by parents. "Go to your room" or "stand in the corner" are examples. There are two general ways in which this procedure can be used.

With the first method, a time out area would be designated (e.g., a room, a corner, the hall) and the child sent there for a particular behavior. For example, every time a child whines he would be sent to the time out area. This type of punishment could be used for temper tantrums, sassiness, fighting between siblings, and numerous other behaviors. The second method involves taking time out from a pleasurable activity. For example, a child may be swimming and may keep going by the forbidden deep end of the pool. Using time out the parent would tell the child, "If you go by the deep end again, you will have to get out of the pool for five minutes." Another situation where this could be used would be where two brothers are watching cartoons. You know they love the cartoons, but they are constantly arguing and fighting with each other. You might tell them, "If I hear any fighting the TV will be turned off for five minutes." The activity from which the child is required to take time out could be anything that is important to him or her (e.g., riding his bike, watching TV, playing with her friends).

Several things must be kept in mind to make this technique successful. First, it has to be very clear what the child needs to do to be punished—the behavior has to be defined and spelled out. For example, the parent may say, "I don't want to hear or see any more fighting. By that I mean hitting each other, name calling, and teasing." This way the child knows exactly what behaviors will be followed by time out. Next, some type of warning should be given. "The next time I see you do that you will have to go to your room" or "I'm going to count to three, and if the fighting does not stop the TV will be turned off." The third thing to keep in mind is that the child should know how long he will be in time out or what she must do to get out of the time out area. For example, "Go to your room for five minutes. I'm going to set the timer on the stove and when the bell rings you can come out." A child who is having a temper tantrum or being sassy might be told, "Go to your room and when you calm down or can talk to me in a normal tone you can come out."

The time out procedure has to be used consistently and may have to be employed several times to control the behavior. The parent whose children are watching the cartoons and fighting may have to turn the TV off for five minutes seven or eight times during the course of the morning. Finally, time out should be given in a very matter-of-fact way without emotion. When you bring the child to time out or when he or she is in the time out area, you should not lecture, scold, or apologize.

Withholding Reward

When a reward system is used and the child does not receive the positive consequence, this can be viewed as a type of punishment. Often, when I am designing a technique using reward to change a behavior, parents ask me, "If she doesn't do what we want her to do, how do we punish her?" My answer is "You don't have to punish her. Not receiving the reward can serve as the negative consequence." For example, consider a child who teases his sister and eventually makes her whine and cry. He loves to stay up past his bedtime and is told, "If you and your sister get along from dinner to bedtime, you can stay up thirty minutes past your bedtime." When he does not comply, he does not necessarily have to be punished. Not receiving the reward is often an effective disciplinary tactic.

Some parents have a hard time accepting that punishment is not always necessary. This is similar to the way most of us are disciplined regarding attendance at work. If you go to work, you are paid, but if you stay home you receive less on payday. We are not punished for missing work. We just do not receive the positive consequence or reward, and this is sufficient to keep most of us going to work on a regular basis.

Verbal Punishment

Hollering, screaming, criticizing, name calling, and lectures, as well as telling the child things to make him or her feel guilty, embarrassed, or fearful are in the category of verbal punishment. This is a very ineffective form of punishment because some children totally ignore their parents' ranting and raving. It goes in one ear and out the other. Still other children have emotional difficulties or behavior problems as a result of verbal punishment. Some children develop resentment and anger toward their parents when this is used; others become emotionally distant.

Most of the possible problems that may occur when punishment is used as the main form of discipline can result from frequent use of verbal punishment. Negative verbal discipline should be avoided.

Physical Punishment

Spanking, whipping, slapping, and hitting children constitute physical punishment. I personally feel that numerous other forms of discipline can be used with children and that this form of punishment should be used very, very sparingly. Parents serve as primary models, and children who receive physical discipline often learn aggressive methods to control others. Other children withdraw, become angry, develop rebellious tendencies, or show a variety of emotional or behavioral difficulties when this type of consequence is employed.

If this form of punishment is used, it should be infrequent and only for certain behaviors. That is, a child should not get a whipping for hitting his sister, getting a detention, coming home late, breaking a toy, and forty other behaviors. Spanking should be reserved for certain behaviors and only used in those cases. This type of punishment is more effective when used with younger children (under four years of age). For example, a small child may get a spanking for crossing the street unattended or for fooling with an electrical outlet, but not for hundreds of different behaviors ranging from wetting his pants to hitting her baby sister.

In addition, some parents should not use physical punishment because it does not fit their personalities. That is, the whipping upsets them more than the child—they feel guilty, mean, or unfair.

QUESTIONS ABOUT PUNISHMENT

How Much Punishment Should Be Given? This is a question I am frequently asked; what most parents mean by it is, "How much should I take away?" "How severe or harsh should the punishment be?" "Should I take him off the baseball team or just not let him ride his bike?" and so forth. This is a difficult question to answer mainly because it depends on the individual children, but several general points can be made.

One of the main factors that control or change behavior is *not* large or severe consequences that occur every now and then, but the small consequences that follow a response each time it is made. For example, why do you avoid touching fire? Probably *not* because you think you will die, get third-degree burns, or have to be hospitalized. The main reason you avoid this behavior is because every time you touch fire or something hot it hurts.

Let's say a child is not doing all of his homework because he is "forgetting" some of his books at school. You have been telling him for three weeks to bring all of his books home, but this is not working. You finally reach the end of your rope and tell him, "If you do not bring all your books home, I will have to take you off the football team"—a pretty significant punishment because this child lives for football. However, the behavior does not change, and he is not allowed to play on the team. Usually in cases of severe punishment the child feels "what's the use"; in the above example he would probably not bring home any books after being punished in this fashion.

A better way to handle this situation would be to identify something important to the child that can occur each time books are left at school. Suppose you are using a response cost system and this child loves to watch TV (it could be any other privilege that is important to him). He is told, "Every time you do not bring all your books home you will lose your TV privileges for that night. So, if you want to watch TV all you have to do is bring your books home." Each time he fails to do as told this consequence would follow.

How Long Should Punishment Last? This also is a frequently asked question and involves similar principles to those discussed above. The important thing to keep in mind is: the closer the punishment occurs to the inappropriate behavior, the greater the effect.

I am sure that we all have experienced this: A child misbehaves and you send her to her room for an hour. She goes, and for about the first five or ten minutes lays on her bed and pouts, complains, or cries. However, after a short period of time, she gets a toy and starts playing with it, reads a book, or occupies herself in some other fashion. With the exception of a brief period of time in the beginning of the punishment, it appears that this does not bother her. Another example would be taking a child's bike away for two weeks for some undesirable behavior. During the first day or so the child is concerned about the punishment, he does not like what has happened, and asks to ride his bike. After the brief period of time in the beginning, it seems as if he could care less about not being able to ride his bike.

In both of the above examples, the probable reason for the "I don't care" attitude about the punishment was that it was too long. Negative consequences do not have to last a long time to work. In fact, the most effective part of any negative consequence occurs in the beginning. Table 5-1 will demonstrate this point.

TABLE 5-1. Length and Effectiveness of Punishments

Effect on behavior	90%	8%	2%	0%	0%	0%
Time in room	10 min	20 min	30 min	40 min	50 min	60 min

Let's take an example of sending a child to his room for one hour for being sassy. In the table you can see that the first ten minutes have a 90 percent effect on the sassiness, the second ten-minute period 8 percent, and the third ten-minute period 2 percent. The punishment has no impact on the behavior during the remaining three ten-minute blocks of time. The latter part of the punishment is very ineffective; during this time the child occupies himself with other things or develops anger and resentment toward the parent. Rather than sending the child to his room one time for an hour, it would be much more effective if he were sent to his room for ten minutes on six different occasions. That is, if he is sassy he goes to his room for ten minutes and then comes out. When this behavior is seen again, the same consequence occurs, and so forth. The same principles would apply in the example of taking a child's bike away for two weeks. Rather than taking the privilege away one time for fourteen days, it would be better to restrict the child for one day fourteen times.

Because children's estimates of time are greatly different from those of adults, punishing a child for one hour might be equivalent to punishing an adult for eight hours. This is particularly true for children with short attention spans or other overactive characteristics. As children get older their perception of time gradually comes to approximate that of an adult. For some small children a thirty-second time out punishment would be sufficient, while for older children twenty minutes may be necessary.

One good rule of thumb to keep in mind when determining how long to punish your child is to watch her closely and see how she reacts. See how long it takes before she occupies herself with something and appears to care less about the punishment. In the above example of sending a child to her room for one hour, we observed whining, complaining, crying, or similar behaviors during the first ten minutes and hardly any reaction to the punishment during the remaining fifty minutes. Therefore, we have some idea of how long to punish the next time—ten minutes. For the child who had his bike taken away for two weeks, we noticed that it

86

affected him the first day and apparently had little impact on his attitude after that. Therefore, one day may be more appropriate the next time this punishment is employed.

MAKING PUNISHMENT EFFECTIVE

Punishment is a consequence that can be used to change behavior. However, several things must be kept in mind to make punishment work effectively and to minimize problems.

Use Punishment with Other Consequences

Punishment is more effective when the other consequences, ignoring and especially reward, are used. When punishment is used as the main method of control, it will be less effective than when used in conjunction with reward. Reward and ignoring should be used about 60 percent to 70 percent of the time, with punishment being utilized 30 percent to 40 percent of the time. Time out and response cost punishment will be more effective if the child is earning rewards and privileges for other behaviors.

Often it is necessary to point out a child's mistakes, especially when teaching new behaviors, but if that is all that is done correction will fall on a deaf ear. Criticism will be significantly more effective if it is sandwiched with praise and emphasis on good behavior. Let's say you ask a child to make her bed for the first time, and after she completes the task you only point out the mistakes. Bed making will become a negative experience, she will avoid it, and your attempts to teach this task will be minimized. However, if you go in after she has made the bed and accentuate all of her successes and the positive points of this behavior and sneak in some criticism every now and then, she is apt to learn more and incorporate your correction into her next attempt at bed making.

The more reward, praise, and positive attention are used, the more effective the punishment system will be.

Define Behaviors and Consequences Clearly

Parents should try to avoid ambiguous statements such as "be good," and state exactly what they mean by being good. "We are going to the store, and I want you to stay by me and not run all over." Spell out the negative consequence along with the rule before misbehavior occurs. For example, "We are going to the store, and if you stay by me you can go outside and play when we get home. If you run all over and do not listen to me, you will have to stay inside when we get home."

Let the Child Know
How to Get out of the Punishment

For many children parents say, "Go to your room," and "You can't ride your bike," or something similar. Then the child asks "For how long?" and the parent says, "When I decide to let you out" or "When I think you deserve to ride your bike." When a child is punished he should know for how long or what he has to do to get out of the punishment. For example, "Go to your room for five minutes." "If you leave your bike in front of the house, you won't be able to ride it tomorrow."

Avoid Punishing a Behavior the First Time,
Use It to Set a Rule

This principle can be employed in the majority of situations. For example, a few days ago I went into my backyard and found some of my tools in the grass starting to rust. I was angry and called my two boys to ask who did this. They both confessed, and I felt like setting down some punishment for this behavior. However, punishment in this situation would be ineffective. It would not change the behavior significantly, because this is a new behavior and the consequences were not spelled out ahead of time. A better way to deal with this situation would be to use it to set the ground rules. For example, "I do not want you going in the garage and playing with my tools or leaving them outside. The next time this happens, you will not be able to look at TV that night."

Use Warnings or Signals

Often a child has to be told over and over again. Each time the parent's voice gets louder and louder, and eventually the parent starts screaming. Only then does the child run and pick up the toys. The child is responding to signals. He waits for the signal that comes before the consequences and then responds. That is, he knows that screaming comes right before punishment is going to happen. Therefore, when these signals appear he performs the desired behavior to avoid the negative consequence. The use of appropriate signals and warnings can make things run more smoothly and eliminate a significant amount of the hassle at home.

Events in the environment can serve as signals. "I want the garbage put out after we eat dinner." "The toys have to be picked up before this TV program is over." "Come home when the street lights come on." You can let events or clues in the environment warn the child and not your voice.

Counting to three, giving three warnings holding up one finger at a time, saying "The next time that happens," or some other very matter-of-fact verbal statement can also serve as effective signals. For example, every time the phone rings and a mother starts talking, her young child creates a series of interruptions—"Let me talk. Where's my ball? I'm thirsty"—the conversation is interrupted, and the parent gradually loses her patience. The mother could use hand signals. The rules, behavioral expectations, and consequences would be set up ahead of time and the child told, "When the phone rings, I don't want you to interrupt me. [What this means should be explained in detail to the child.] Each time you interrupt me I'm going to hold up a finger, and if I get to three fingers, you will have to go to your room for five minutes" or some similar punishment. Reward could also be used. "If I don't get to three warnings, I'll read you a story." Pennies, pencils, or some other object could be placed on a table as signals. The child would be told, "Each time you interrupt me I'm going to take a penny off the table. When there are no pennies left, you'll have to go to your room for five minutes." You have to be consistent when using this type of warning system and give the third or final warning when appropriate. You cannot say, "I'm going to count to three. One . . . two . . . two . . . two." And three never comes.

Using signals to create a buffer period may also reduce some behavioral problems. Suppose you are watching a suspense movie on TV and you are about to find out who is guilty of the murder, when your spouse asks you to go to the kitchen and get him or her a drink. What would you say? "Wait till this program's over" because you are involved in what is happening, you have been waiting two hours for this moment. We do this to our children frequently. For example, a child is outside playing baseball, it is almost her turn to bat, and her mother says, "Come in, it's time to eat." In this situation you get a lot of resistance from the child. Often this could be avoided by giving the child a five-minute warning. A little while before it would be time to come in you would say, "I'm going to call you in five minutes to come in. Start getting ready. The next time I call you, come in." In other words, sometimes it is not wise to demand that a child do what you expect at that minute. Give a signal to serve as a buffer period and reduce some of the resistance.

Individualized Punishment

When deciding on a negative consequence, the interests, values, and preferences of the child must be considered. What may be punishing for one child may not be negative for another. For some children going to their room is a major punishment, but others could care less. Parents may tell their child, "If you don't get dressed on time for school, you will miss the bus and will not be able to go to school."Some children would consider this a negative consequence, others would see it as a reward.

Punish the Behavior, Not the Child

You have probably heard Joyce Brothers say this many times. I like you as an individual, but your behavior is unacceptable. When you use punishment you should comment on the behavior and not on the child as an individual. If a child fails a test in school, this does not mean he is stupid (a statement concerning a child's self-image). It means that he did not adequately study for the test. If a child is hitting her brother, she is not necessarily a mean person. However, this type of behavior may not be tolerated.

Stay Calm When Punishing

Whenever punishment is administered, you should remain calm, cool, and collected. The behavior being dealt with should be treated in a matter-of-fact fashion. If a child loses a privilege (response cost) or is put in a time out area, avoid nagging, scolding, or lecturing.

Assign Punishments for Specific Behaviors

Parents often use the same negative consequence for many different behaviors. When this is done, punishment loses its effectiveness as a motivator for behavior change. In using negative consequences, specific punishments should be used for specific behaviors. Use loss of TV time only when certain behaviors are seen (e.g., homework is not completed or sassiness). Physical punishment or going to your room should be related to specific actions. By doing this you can avoid the problems that occur when negative consequences are overused.

Administer Punishment Immediately

The importance or effectiveness of punishment, like that of reward, is primarily determined by how close it occurs to the behavior you are trying to control or change and *not* by its severity, length, or harshness. Therefore, the statement "You must make the punishment fit the crime" is not always true. However, the statement "Punishment should occur as soon as reasonably possible after the misbehavior" is very accurate.

Negative consequences have the most impact on the behaviors that occur right before the punishment. Let's say right after school a brother and sister get into a fight. Mother comes in, separates the children, and says, "Wait till your dad gets home, you both will be punished." About three hours pass and the children are playing together and having a good time. The father comes home and the mother relates the incident that occurred earlier. Dad gives the children a lecture and administers a punishment.

Children's conception of time is different from ours. A six-year-old child may perceive fifteen minutes like we perceive two hours. Therefore, if the consequence is too far removed from the behavior, he may not remember why he is being punished.

chapter six

IGNORING OR NO CONSEQUENCES

Some behaviors in children exist because of the reaction given to them by their parents. Some kids know that whining, complaining, pouting, sassiness, temper outbursts, or crying will get a reaction from their parents and will get them their way. Behaviors similar to these are often maintained because of the consequences children receive for them. All behavior exists for a reason, and to eliminate some types of child behavior, it is necessary to remove the consequence. That is, ignore the behavior. Ignoring undesirable actions is a very powerful method of discipline, but it is not often effectively used by most parents.

Ignoring or providing no consequence only changes or eliminates certain behaviors. For others, it has no effect. The obvious question is "What should be ignored?" You should *not* ignore behaviors that are task oriented, that is, actions that perform a duty, disrupt the activities of others, or may lead to injury to others or damage to property. For example, making your bed, taking your bath, doing your homework, cleaning up your room, hitting your sister, breaking a glass, or similar behaviors should not be ignored. Positive or negative consequences should be employed to deal with these.

To determine what behaviors should be ignored, you should analyze the action and ask, "What is the child getting out of the behavior?" If the answer is: "He's getting me upset," "she's making me holler and scream," "we get into a power struggle or screaming match," or "I give in to her," then this is the type of behavior that should be ignored.

Let's say you ask your child to put out the garbage. While he is doing what you requested, he starts mumbling under his breath. Most of it cannot be understood, but every now and then you hear something like "They think I'm a slave around here. They always make me do stuff, my brother never has to do anything." Although he is putting out the garbage as you have asked him, you start reacting to the mumbling—"Speak up. What are you saying? You better cut that out. Stop mumbling"—and each time your voice is getting louder and you are becoming more and more upset.

Probably the main reason this child's mumbling continues is your reaction to it. Therefore, it should be ignored. A similar situation occurs when you send a child to her room. She goes to her room and starts making noises, telling you how mean you are, hitting the wall, singing at the top of her voice. If the behavior is ignored and the child does not get a response, the behavior usually disappears because it serves no purpose.

Behaviors that are manipulative (e.g., whining, pouting, temper tantrums), should also be ignored. A child says, "Can I go outside and play?" It is almost time to eat so you say, "No." This brings a violent reaction from the child. He starts screaming and throws himself on the floor. After a little while you cannot take it any more so you tell him, "Go outside and play. I'll call you when it is time to eat." Often children can wear down their parents with continuous whining, pleading, and other behaviors and finally get their way.

TYPES OF IGNORING RESPONSES

Ignoring these types of behavior usually produce behavioral change, but this has to be employed consistently. There are two general ways to provide no consequences to a specific behavior in a child.

Withdraw All Attention
Pretend the behavior does not exist or the child is not there. You should not talk to the child, make facial or gestural indications

of disapproval, or mumble to yourself—withdraw all attention. If you decide to ignore whining and the child exhibits this behavior while you are talking to someone, simply talk over the behavior. Turning up the TV, putting on the stereo headset, going outside to work in the garden, taking a walk, or becoming involved with a task are some techniques you can use to help withdraw all attention from the misbehavior.

Withdraw Emotional Attention,
But Deal with the Behavior
With this type of ignoring the screaming, verbal reprimands, and emotional attention by the parent are eliminated, but some disciplinary action, usually time out or response cost punishment, is taken. For example, the rule at your house may be, "When someone has a temper tantrum he goes to his room. When he calms down, he can come out." Therefore, when a child throws a temper tantrum, simply tell her to go to her room or bring her there. Do not get upset, tell her to stop, or threaten a whipping.

Sassiness may be dealt with by stating, "I will not talk to you when you are sassy." (You would explain exactly what you mean by this.) When the child starts being sassy, you would emotionally ignore it and state, "When you can talk in a normal tone of voice, I will respond to you."

MAKING IGNORING EFFECTIVE

When ignoring is used to manage overactive behaviors, certain things must be kept in mind.

Be Consistent
It is extremely important to be consistent when this disciplinary consequence is chosen to deal with a behavior. If you choose to ignore pouting, you must do it every time the behavior occurs. You cannot ignore it one time and attend to it the next, because if the child wins (i.e., gets what he or she wants from the behavior) every now and then, this may be sufficient to keep the behavior going. By being inconsistent, you set up a situation for the child similar to

that of a gambler. That is, he may lose seven or ten times, but win once; this one win is enough to keep him trying fifteen more times.

Be Sure the Behavior Is Actually Being Ignored

Many times parents think they are ignoring a behavior, but they are not totally eliminating all attention or consequences. Therefore, be sure that *all* verbal (e.g., lecturing, hollering, mumbling under your breath) and nonverbal (e.g., angry expression on your face, slamming a door) communications are withdrawn from the child's undesirable behavior.

Be Prepared for the Behavior to Get Worse

Sometimes when the attention or consequences that are usually given a behavior are withdrawn, the behavior will intensify before it gets better. Think of a child who has temper tantrums and usually gets his way. It usually takes a five-minute tantrum to get to his parents enough for them to give in to his desires. Now the parents have attended one of our workshops and they are going to stick to what they say and ignore the behavior. The child comes in and asks his mother, "Can I have a Coke?" She says, "No, you have already had two." The temper tantrum starts; at the end of five minutes the parent has not attended to this behavior and has not given in. What is going to happen now that he has not received the consequences he usually gets? The behavior is going to intensify. His voice may get louder. The crying may occur more frequently, and the length of the temper tantrum will increase. It may last ten, thirty, or sixty minutes, or until the child realizes the behavior is not going to bring him the consequence he normally receives. The behavior is not working, and the only things the temper tantrum gets him are an upset stomach, sore throat, and a headache. Therefore, it serves no purpose and should stop or start decreasing in frequency and intensity.

Something we are all familiar with can illustrate these points. Suppose you walk up to a soft drink machine, deposit your money, make your selection, and nothing happens (the machine ignores you). The usual behavior that gets you the desired consequence does not work. What would you do? You would start pressing the coin return and selection buttons, and if the machine continues to ignore you, your behavior would increase in frequency. If these attempts are unsuccessful, you would probably start hitting or kicking the machine. After a while, you might stop and rest and try it again. But this time you will not try as hard or as long. This may be done several times, but each time the intensity and frequency of the behavior will decrease. If the machine continues to ignore you and you are unsuccessful in getting the drink or your money back, you will give up these actions because they are useless. Your behavior changes; you either walk away or tell someone that you lost your money.

The same thing happens when this consequence is used to deal with whining, complaining, pouting, noise making, and similar behaviors. The behavior intensifies or increases in frequency until the child realizes it is not serving a purpose, and then it will start to disappear. For example, if a child whines about five times a day, about ten minutes each time, and is ignored, the periods of whining may increase and the behavior may be seen more than five times a day. However, if the parent hangs in and keeps ignoring the behavior, the length of the whining periods will get shorter and the number of times the behavior will be seen each day will decrease. The child will periodically test the parent to see if the parent will still stick to his guns until he realizes the behavior is fruitless. Then he will change his behavior and the whining will be eliminated. Therefore, when the behavior gets worse it is important that you continue doing the same thing, do not give in, and do not go back to your old methods of dealing with the undesirable behavior. The increase in the inappropriate behavior should last three to five days at most. In the majority of situations, the increase will last only one or two days.

If the above procedures are accurately employed, the most severe temper tantrums and other similar behaviors can be successfully dealt with in a few days.

Use Ignoring Initially, but Employ Other
Consequences to Change Behavior
For the types of behaviors described in this chapter, a good rule to keep in mind is to try the consequence of ignoring first. This disciplinary tactic will usually produce successful results on behaviors whose primary purpose is to get a reaction from the parent

or to get the child what he or she wants. However, in some cases ignoring the behavior will not be sufficient to change it. In these situations, positive or negative consequences must be employed when the ignored behavior does not improve.

Ignore the Reactions of Others

When this consequence is being used and other people are around (e.g., at a store, company at home), some parents may feel embarrassed or pressured into some action that will counteract what they are trying to accomplish. Try to disregard the reactions of others and how you think they perceive you—deal with your child's behavior and not other people.

chapter seven
BEHAVIOR CHARTS

Behavior charts are often very helpful in dealing with an overactive child's behavior. They not only provide a formal record of the child's behavior, but also add structure and predictability to the environment.

SETTING UP A BEHAVIOR CHART

ANALYZE THE BEHAVIOR

The first step in developing a chart is to analyze the target behavior. How frequently does it occur? Under what circumstances is the behavior seen? How long does it last? Analysis is very important, because it will primarily determine what type of chart will be constructed.

IDENTIFY AN IMPORTANT CONSEQUENCE

Whether reward or punishment is used, the next step would be to select a consequence that is important to the child. Most charts are based on reward and are set up in positive terms for the reasons discussed in Chapters 4 and 5. However, a behavior chart also lends itself easily to a response cost system of discipline.

TYPES OF BEHAVIOR CHARTS

The number and style of behavior charts available to parents are only limited by their imagination. I will describe several general types.

BEHAVIOR OCCURS OR CAN OCCUR MORE THAN ONCE A DAY

Sometimes the behavior you are trying to change is seen many times through the day (e.g., not listening, stubbornness, whining). In this situation two options are available. One chart could be based on time periods or how often the behavior is seen. The other would be based on frequency or how many times a day the behavior occurs.

Time Periods

Suppose the target behavior is stubbornness. You have analyzed the behavior and found it an average of about seven times a day. You have decided to construct a chart by breaking the day up into time periods. The chart might look similar to Chart 7-1.

	Monday	Tuesday	Wednesday	Thursday	Friday	Saturday	Sunday
Before School	★	X	X	★	X	X	★
3 – 5 o'clock	X	★	★	X	★	★	★
5 – 7 o'clock	X	X	X	X	★	★	★
7 – Bedtime	X	X	★	X	X	X	★

Chart 7.1. Ben's Cooperation Chart (First Week)

You divide the week into days and the days into four time periods. A reward has been identified: let's say five minutes past bedtime. You then tell the child, "For each period of time that passes when you have cooperated with me [explain what you mean by this], I will put a star on your chart. When you are stubborn [explain what you mean by this] during a period of time, I will put an X in that block. At the end of each day, you can trade in each star you have for five minutes past your bedtime. Do you understand what I've said? Explain what I said in your own words." If the child understands the system, start. If not, reexplain it.

If you have a timer on your stove or a cooking timer, set it for the time period. When the bell rings, calmly mark an X if the child has been stubborn during that time, or you could put the X when the behavior occurs. If he has been cooperative, affix a star and give the child verbal or social reward (praise him for his good behavior). Then reset the timer and follow the same procedure again.

Depending on the age of the child, the behavior you are trying to change, and whether you have previously used charts, the reward could be given several ways.

1. After each time period: When a child receives a star during a time period he would be rewarded immediately (e.g., a piece of candy, a story read to him).
2. Daily: At the end of each day the child could trade in her stars for a reward (e.g., five minutes past her bedtime for each star. If she has two stars, her parents will play a game with her).
3. Weekly: At the end of the week he could trade in his stars for a reward (e.g., twelve stars earn a trip to the park, movie, or whatever on Saturday or Sunday).
4. Every other week, once a month, or less often.

The most important aspect of reward or punishment is how close it occurs to the target behavior. Therefore, for overactive children with short attention spans, or when you first start using charts with children, the time before they receive the reward should be minimal.

Let's say you are analyzing another behavior (e.g., bossing other children) and find that it occurs very frequently, an average of twenty times a day. You would construct a similar chart, but the time periods would be much smaller, possibly every half hour (see Chart 7-2).

With this chart, the child would have to earn more tokens to receive the same reward as in Chart 7-1. For example, under this system one star may represent two minutes past her bedtime or she may have to earn forty stars to get a trip to the park. As the child starts receiving more stars each week, the time periods would

	Monday	Tuesday	Wednesday	Thursday	Friday	Saturday	Sunday
7:30 – 8:00	X	X	★	★	★	★	★
8:00 – 8:30	★	X	★	★	★	X	★
3:30 – 4:00	★	X	★	X	★	★	★
4:00 – 4:30	X	★	★	X	★	★	★
4:30 – 5:00	X	★	X	★	★	★	X
5:00 – 5:30	★	★	X	★	★	★	X
5:30 – 6:00	X	X	X	★	X	★	X
6:30 – 7:00	★	X	★	★	X	★	★
7:00 – 7:30	★	★	★	X	★	★	★
7:30 – 8:00	X	★	X	X	★	★	★
8:00 – 8:30	★	★	X	X	★	★	★
8:30 – 9:00	★	★	★	★	★	★	★

Chart 7.2. Val's Getting Along with Others Chart (First Week)

be increased—say to every hour. As the child improves, the day might be broken up into four blocks of time like in Chart 7-1.

As you use the chart and the child improves, the amount of stars he or she has to earn each week to receive the reward is increased. For example, during the second week in Chart 7-1, the child would have to earn fifteen stars to go to the park, the third week he would need seventeen stars to go to a movie, and so forth.

Frequency of Behavior

Suppose you analyze a behavior (e.g., not listening) and find out that it occurs more than once a day. You decide to construct a chart based on frequency or how many times a day the behavior occurs—let's say an average of ten times a day (see Chart 7-3).

You have divided the week up into days and put ten circles on each day (the not listening occurs an average of that many times a day). Next, you identify an important reward or punishment. Using a reward system, you would tell the child, "I'm putting ten circles on each day of the week. Each time you do not listen [explain exactly what you mean by this], I am going to go to your chart and color in one of those circles."

If you're using a daily reward system, you would tell him,

Monday	Tuesday	Wednesday	Thursday	Friday	Saturday	Sunday
● ●	● ●	● ●	● ●	● ●	○ ○	○ ○
● ●	● ●	● ●	● ●	● ●	○ ○	○ ○
● ●	● ★	● ●	★ ★	★ ★	○ ○	○ ○
● ★	★ ★	● ★	★ ★	★ ★	○ ○	○ ○
★ ★	★ ★	★ ★	★ ★	★ ★	○ ○	○ ○

Chart 7.3. Jeffrey's Listening Chart (First Week)

"At the end of the day we will go to your chart and you will put a star on every circle that is not colored. You can trade your stars in for the reward [something that has already been determined]." If you are using a weekly reward system, the stars would be traded in at the end of the week instead of daily.

Using a response cost system of punishment on a daily basis, you would tell the child, "At the end of the day we will go to your chart and count the colored-in circles. For each colored circle you will lose ten minutes of TV time" or whatever has been predetermined. If you are using a weekly punishment system, you would tell him, "If you have thirty-five colored-in circles by the weekend you will lose this privilege [any consequence that was considered important]."

When frequency is used as the basis of constructing a behavior chart, another type could be also developed. Suppose you have a child who never picks up her clothes or toys even after she has been told to do so. You have analyzed the behavior and found it to occur about seven times a day. You might set up a chart similar to Chart 7-4.

You have divided the week up into days, but have left each one blank. You then identify a reward. Next you tell the child, "Each time I ask you to pick up something [explain what you mean by this] and you do it the first time I ask you, I will put a star on the chart. If I have to remind you more than once, you will not get a star." Then at the end of the day, week, or whatever she would be able to trade in her stars for the reward.

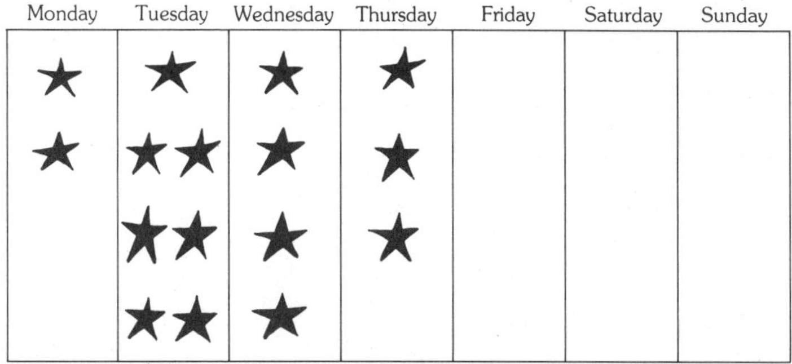

Chart 7.4. Julie's Pickup Chart (First Week)

When working to change a behavior that occurs more than once a day, do *not* include more than one behavior on the chart. If you want to work on another behavior, another chart should be constructed. However, it is best not to have more than two charts going at one time. Wait till the child's sassiness has significantly improved, then substitute another behavior of concern.

BEHAVIOR OCCURS OR CAN OCCUR ONLY ONCE A DAY

If you are concerned with a behavior that is seen infrequently or can occur only once a day (e.g., getting dressed for school, taking a bath, homework), the charts described above would not be appropriate. In these situations two different approaches could be used: verbal or written contracts and formal charts.

Verbal Agreement

This is usually used for only one behavior at a time. The child would be told, "On the days that you get dressed for school on time you can have an extra dime to take to school. On the days that you are late you get the amount you usually receive." The child would then be asked to repeat the verbal agreement to be sure that he or she understands it correctly.

Another example would be, "If you bring all your books home from school, you can stay up past your bedtime. If not, you go to bed at the usual time."

Written Contract

For some children a verbal contract is not sufficient. Either they forget it, do not remember all of it, or disagree with the terms once they have not lived up to their part of the agreement. In these situations it is best to formalize the contract in writing. Two examples follow.

Date ________________

When I do my homework without a hassle, I will be able to have a snack at night. When I cause trouble, there will be no snack.

Signed ________________

Signed ________________

Date ________________

I agree to come in from playing when called. If I do, I will be able to stay up thirty minutes past my bedtime. If I do not, I go to bed at the usual time.

Signed ________________

Signed ________________

The agreement is spelled out on paper, and both the parent and the child sign it. Then it is placed conspicuously on the refrigerator or the door to the child's room.

Formal Chart

When a behavior only occurs once a day, the chart can and should include more than one target behavior, but no more than three or four (see Chart 7-5).

Three target behaviors are specified. Because the behaviors only pertain to school, the chart is based on five days instead of seven. The child is then told how he can earn stars and X's, as well as what the stars represent and when they can be traded in (the same procedure as used in Charts 7-1 to 7-4).

	Monday	Tuesday	Wednesday	Thursday	Friday
Getting dressed for school	X	X	★	X	★
Bring all books from school	★	★	★	X	★
Homework without a hassel	X	X	★	★	★

Chart 7.5. Tony's Chart (First Week)

Three unrelated behaviors could also be included on this type of chart (see Chart 7-6).

Household duties and chores could also be included, as in Chart 7-7.

	Monday	Tuesday	Wednesday	Thursday	Friday	Saturday	Sunday
Brushing Teeth	X	X	☺	☺	☺	☺	☺
Taking Bath	☺	☺	☺	X	☺	☺	☺
Going to bed when told	☺	X	☺	X	X	☺	☺

Chart 7.6. Lori's Chart (First Week)

Chart 7.7 Jason's Duties

	Monday	Tuesday	Wednesday	Thursday	Friday	Saturday	Sunday
Making bed	☺	☺	☺	☺	☺	☺	☺
Feeding dog	☺	☺	X	☺	X	☺	X
Cleaning up after dinner	X	X	☺	☺	X	☺	☺

There are many variations on these themes. Generally, behavior charts work better for younger children (ten years old and under), but I have used them with high-school students. The procedures and principles are the same for all age groups, the consequences differ.

WHY USE BEHAVIOR CHARTS?

There are several advantages to using behavior charts.

Charts Provide Immediate Consequences.
Behavior charts help parents deal with the behavior almost immediately. Although the reward will be given at night (e.g., staying up past the child's bedtime), it can be meaningfully represented immediately with a star or an X at 9:00 A.M. A consequence that will occur on Saturday (e.g., a movie, a fishing trip) can be signified on a daily or hourly basis.

In addition, charts help parents break down "big" consequences. For example, your child comes to you and says, "Mike got a new pair of tennis shoes, and I want some like his." You look at his old shoes and he needs a new pair, but you also realize that this could be used as a reward. However, the reward is too "big" to be used for a one-time behavior (e.g., "If you clean your room, we'll go get the shoes"). So, you could construct a chart like Chart 7-8 and have the child earn the shoes with appropriate behaviors over a one-week or two-week period.

Chart 7.8. Alan's Be Good Chart

	Monday	Tuesday	Wednesday	Thursday	Friday	Saturday	Sunday
Before School	X	★	★	X	★	★	★
3 – 5 o'clock	X	★	X	X	★	X	★
5 – 7 o'clock	★	X	★	★	★	★	X
7 – Bedtime	★	X	★	★	★	★	X

12 stars = tennis shoes

Suppose the target behavior is temper tantrums. You would explain the chart and how the stars could be earned and then tell the child, "When Saturday comes, if you have twelve stars we will go get the tennis shoes. If you don't, we'll start over next week. Therefore, we can get the tennis shoes this Saturday or any Saturday in 1985. It's up to you." "Big" punishments or loss of privileges (e.g., not being able to go on a camping trip or not being allowed to spend the weekend at a friend's house) could be dealt with in a similar fashion.

Although the reward or punishment may be received in the future, behavior charts bridge the gap between the occurrence of the behavior and the consequence, thereby helping parents employ immediacy of consequences.

Parents Can Look at Behavior Objectively

PARENT: My children can never get along. They fight continuously. It is driving me crazy. It seems like I'm always correcting them for this.

PSYCHOLOGIST: We can set up a behavior chart to deal with their fighting. [This procedure is then described in detail to the parent.]

Two weeks later.

PSYCHOLOGIST: How did that chart work with your two children? Did the fighting decrease?

PARENT: You know, once we started charting the behavior we realized that it was not as bad as we thought it was. It did not occur nearly as much as we described last time, and now we do not feel it is a problem. Let's focus on something else.

Charting behavior also helps parents see gradual improvement easily. Parents often look at a child's overall behavior and cannot see gradual improvement. For example, we are working on sassy behavior in a child. Parents come in and say, "Our child is very sassy, always has to have the last word, and never has anything nice to say." I outline some techniques for the parents to try. Two weeks later they come back and say, "We've tried what you said, but he's still sassy." If a chart was used we could get an objective look at the behavior and see if any gradual improvement occurred. For example, when we analyzed the behavior we saw that the sassiness occurred an average of ten times a day. During the first week the chart was employed, the target behavior appeared about seven times a day. The behavior decreased to five times a day the second week. Although the child is still sassy, the target behavior has improved significantly, 50 percent, in two weeks.

Problem behaviors do not occur overnight, they gradually develop. Improvement is also gradual, and behavior charts help parents see this.

Charts Help Parents Be Consistent

Consistency is the foundation of effective child management. Charts help parents follow behaviors consistently. A chart will serve as a good reminder, and children often become involved in getting stars and working toward rewards; they are quick to remind parents when they "forget" to mark the chart or total their stars for the day.

Just the Structure Provided by Charts
Is Beneficial for Some Children

The mere facts that a child can see the chart, put stars on it, and become involved in working toward a reward are helpful to some children. The additional structure provided by behavior charts and the subsequent involvement in charting "good" behavior often facilitates positive change in overactive children.

Token Rewards Can Easily Be Used with Charts

Token rewards have little value in themselves, but they represent something important or can be traded in for a desired object. Just as some adults will work to save money and put it in the bank but have no intention of spending it, some children will work just to receive and horde tokens with little intention of trading them. This is especially true after a chart has been used for three or four weeks. The parent might ask the child in the beginning of the week, "What do you want to work for this week?" The child may not be able to identify a specific reward, but will work hard all week. At the end of the week he may have earned enough stars to receive the reward, but not be anxious to trade them in. The tokens themselves serve as the reward.

I have used stars as tokens, but numerous things can be used depending on your imagination. Some parents have used animal shapes, smile faces, gold stars, stickers, and checkmarks. Other parents employ more complex systems, such as different colored stars for different behaviors (e.g., a blue star if a child does not fight with his sister and a red star for not fighting with and not teasing his sister), with each color having a specific trade-in value. Others have used numbers (3 = very good, 2 = pretty good, 1 = good, 0 = not good), with the reward based on a specific point total. Regardless of token used, be sure that the child understands the system and that it is appropriate for and important to him or her.

Positive Behaviors Can Be Emphasized
Charts that focus on positive behaviors (e.g., getting along with your sister, being cooperative, listening) help parents look at the child's "good" behaviors. Therefore, praise and more attention can be given to these appropriate actions.

MAKING BEHAVIOR CHARTS EFFECTIVE

Lock the Child into the System
with Minimal Expectations
When first using a chart the parent should make it somewhat easy for the child to obtain the reward. Once the child is locked into the system, the expectations can be gradually increased. The best way to lose a child's interest in a chart is to have him at first fail to achieve the reward.

PARENT: You know that chart you told us to use to help Joey control his temper? Well, it worked pretty good at first, but now it seems as if he could care less about it. It doesn't seem to make any difference to him whether he gets a star or an X.
PSYCHOLOGIST: Tell me how you designed the chart.
PARENT: We analyzed the behavior and found that he displayed inappropriate anger about ten times a day. We set up the chart like you told us with ten circles on each day [like Chart 7-3]. Each time he lost his temper, we colored in a circle, and at the end of the day we put stars on the circles that were not filled in. However, the first week he did not get

enough stars to obtain the reward. During the second and third weeks, he lost all interest in the chart. What do we do now?

PSYCHOLOGIST: What was the reward and what did he have to do to earn it?

PARENT: If he got forty stars by Saturday (an average of eight a day), he could go to a movie he has been wanting to see real bad. He only got twenty in the five days.

PSYCHOLOGIST: You expected him to change too much, and it was probably too difficult for him to do. Because he failed the first week, the chart became negative, and he lost interest. Remember you told me he was having ten temper outbursts a day. You required him to get eight stars a day to go to the movie. That's an 80 percent improvement in one week. That would be difficult for anybody. Let's look at another thing. He obtained twenty stars, an average of four a day. By not receiving the reward you "punished" him for changing his behavior 40 percent in a week, and this is another reason why he lost interest.

When starting a chart, make the expectations reasonable so the child can achieve the reward. A good rule to keep in mind when beginning a chart is to make the reward dependent on 30 percent to 40 percent improvement. In the above example of ten temper outbursts a day, the child should receive a reward if he reduces the target behavior to an average of six or seven a day and earns three or four stars a day. Each week the chart is employed, the expectations are gradually increased. For example, the second week the child may have to show 45 percent improvement to get the reward, the third week 55 percent, and so forth. But never expect 100 percent improvement for behaviors that occur frequently— always allow some room for error.

Keep the Chart Simple

Do not include too many behaviors on the chart or make it too complex.

One time a parent told me a chart that she was using was not working. I asked her what she had on it. The list below was her response:

1. Get out of bed when called
2. Get dressed for school on time
3. Brush teeth

4. Eat breakfast
5. Put school clothes in dirty clothes basket
6. Do homework
7. Come in from play when told
8. Eat dinner
9. Clean up room
10. Take bath without hassle
11. Go to bed when told

Needless to say, there are too many target behaviors on this chart and two things could happen. First, the child will give up easily or not attempt the behaviors at all. In the above example, the child may have gotten fifteen minutes past his bedtime for all that work and felt it was not worth the effort. In addition, children tend to avoid things that look too big or involve a lot of work. We all do this. If you have a large pile of clothes to wash or a lot of paperwork to do, you are likely to put it off.

Second, when too many behaviors are placed on a chart, the child can easily manipulate the system. That is, she can select certain behaviors to perform, ignore others, and still receive the reward. Usually the behaviors that the child avoids are the most important ones.

If charts are made too complex, the child may become confused about how and when he gets the reward. For example, "A gold star means this, and a blue star represents that. If you have seven by Tuesday, this will happen, but if you have fifteen by Friday, this will also happen. However, you could combine the points you get this week with the ones you get next week, or you could add the ones from last week, or . . ." After all of this, the child is thoroughly confused and says, "Forget about this chart."

Be Sure the Consequences
Earned are Received

PSYCHOLOGIST: Ms. A, tell me about that chart we set up to help your son with his sassiness.

Ms. A: Well, it worked beautifully the first two weeks. He showed about a 90 percent improvement, but the last two weeks he's back to the same old stuff.

Psychologist: What happened? You were doing so well.
        Child: The first week my mother told me that I could go to the
                skating rink Saturday if I earned so many points. I got the
                points I needed, but she said she was too busy to take me.
                The next week was the same thing. I earned the necessary
                points but was not able to go skating. So, I figure what's the
                use?

When this happens you can't expect a chart to work for more than
a short period of time no matter how well it is constructed. Be sure
you keep your end of the contract. If a child earns certain consequences, be sure he receives them.

Make the Chart Positive

Most of the charts I set up involve positive consequences
rather than negative ones. In addition, verbal or social reward
should always be associated with behavior charts. When the child
is placing her token on the chart and when she receives the final
consequence, she should be praised. Descriptions of the target
behaviors should also be stated in a positive manner. Rather than
negative statements like "fighting with your sister," "messy
room," or "coming home late," the descriptions on the charts
should read positively—"getting along with your sister," "cleaning
room," or "coming home on time."

HOW LONG SHOULD A CHART BE USED?

This really depends on the individual child and the type of behaviors you are dealing with. A chart should be used for a
minimum of four or five weeks, but may have to be used longer.
One of the mistakes parents make is to discontinue charts too soon.
Once the chart has been in use for a sufficient time and the child is
responding adequately, it can be phased out. This could be done in
several ways. The child could simply be told that he has done well
and the target behavior is under control. Now, you can use the
chart to work on another behavior. Second, you could start increas-
ing the amount of tokens the child has to earn to receive the reward
and try to get him or her to behave for the token rewards. Then
eventually phase out the entire chart. Another method would be
asking the child if he wanted to continue the chart, provided he is

doing well. In quite a few situations you will notice the child losing interest in the chart, and it can be discontinued. When to stop using a chart is difficult to determine arbitrarily, it depends on the child. However, try to avoid stopping before the new behavior has had a chance to establish itself.

chapter eight

WHAT TO DO IF THE TECHNIQUES DO NOT WORK

If these management suggestions do not decrease the child's overactive behaviors, you should consider several things before employing more specific techniques of management.

ARE YOU USING CONSEQUENCES OTHER THAN PUNISHMENT?

Punishment used as the primary method of control will not alter overactive behavior in some children. In fact, it may make matters worse in some situations. The consequences of rewarding and ignoring behaviors must also be employed.

ARE THE TECHNIQUES BEING USED CONSISTENTLY?

Another reason some techniques do not work is that they are not tried consistently. We try something one day and the next day we do something different. We do not stick with the same technique long enough.

Inconsistency also occurs when parents use the technique but do not employ it every time they should. Suppose a child runs through the house constantly, and you tell him, "Every time you run in the house you're going to have to go to your room for two

114

minutes.'' This procedure might be followed in the morning, but not in the afternoon. The child might go to his room half of the time and the other half the behavior is overlooked. The techniques and consequences must be used and administered consistently.

HAVE YOU GIVEN THE TECHNIQUES A CHANCE TO WORK?

Even if parents are consistent and use the same technique in disciplining, some methods do not work simply because they are not tried long enough. Most behaviors in children will not change overnight. For example, a child has been sassy for ten months. Her parents set up a procedure to deal with this behavior. They use the method very consistently, but after three or four days the child is still sassy, so they discontinue the procedure. A behavior that has existed for several months will not disappear in a few days. Attempts to change behavior must be tried for a week or two, sometimes more, before they can be considered ineffective.

DID YOU LOOK FOR SMALL IMPROVEMENTS?

A lot of the behaviors observed in children can be viewed as habits or responses to the environment; they have gradually developed over a long period of time. When we look at our children's behavior most of us look at overall behavior. We do not look for small improvements. You have to break the behavior up into small steps and look for gradual improvements.

ARE THE CONSEQUENCES BEING USED IMPORTANT TO THE CHILD?

Whether negative or positive consequences are used, you have to be very sure that they are important to the child. If the consequence used is not important or appropriate, it will not serve as a motivator, and the behavior will not change. In determining a reward or a punishment you have to consider the individual child's interests and values and use the consequence that is important to him or her. In addition, children change with time; what may be important this week may not serve as a motivator the next week.

DID YOU CONSISTENTLY EMPLOY THE TECHNIQUES IF THE BEHAVIOR AT FIRST GOT WORSE?

Sometimes when an effective technique is being used the behavior will get worse before it gets better. When parents see the behavior getting worse, they stop using the technique. However, the increase in misbehavior may mean that the disciplinary tactic was working, and the parents should not have given it up.

DID YOU PREVENT THE CHILD FROM MANIPULATING YOU?

Children are good manipulators when it comes to getting out of being disciplined. For example, you tell your child, "You can't go outside until you pick up your toys." He says, "I'm not picking them up, and I didn't want to go outside anyway." You then think, "What do I do now?" The child is starting to manipulate you. It may be true that he is not interested in going outside today, but if you know he likes to go outside and make this rule stick, those toys will eventually get picked up and the procedure will work.

If the answer to some of the above questions is "No," you should use the technique again and try to eliminate the reason it did not work. If you feel that you have successfully implemented the general management techniques described in Part II and the overactive behavior has not improved, you may have to consider one of the specific techniques discussed in Part III.

It is important to exhaust other techniques *before* medication is considered. If nondrug techniques are fully implemented and overactive behaviors continue, medication should be considered to help control the interfering symptoms of overactivity.

III

SPECIFIC MANAGEMENT TECHNIQUES

chapter nine
COUNSELING AND PSYCHOTHERAPY

Counseling or psychotherapy involves consultation with a mental health professional, a psychologist, psychiatrist, or social worker. When trying to locate someone to provide these services, be sure he or she has the proper license or certification and has expertise in the type of counseling or psychotherapy your child needs. Regardless of the discipline of the counselor, select someone who primarily deals with children and is familiar with overactive children.

Counseling is often viewed as a more superficial form of treatment that provides information and advice. It is also seen as educative in the sense that the individual is given information or taught new things that can be applied to his or her life. Psychotherapy is usually seen as a more "in-depth" form of treatment, dealing with inner conflicts, feelings, and emotions. Regardless of the type of treatment, research has shown that this is ineffective in treating overactivity if *only* the child is involved.

For counseling or psychotherapy to work with children, the parents must be involved. If I see a child one hour a week, his parents have him the other 167 hours. Therefore, if I can provide the parents with effective methods to deal with the child the rest of the week, the probability of success in changing the child's behavior will greatly increase. In a sense, the parents become the child's "therapists." Counseling and psychotherapy should be primarily geared toward the parents when dealing with overactivity. This is not because the parents are "crazy," "sick," or doing everything wrong, but because they are with the child more. If they have specific techniques to deal with the child's behavior, change will occur faster. Several forms of counseling and psychotherapy are beneficial to overactive children.

PARENTAL COUNSELING

Parental counseling provides suggestions and methods to deal with their child's behavior. The therapist usually gives the parents some general suggestions and works with them on specific behavioral concerns. This kind of treatment is beneficial to all types of overactive children.

PARENTAL WORKSHOPS OR MEETINGS

These are very similar to parental counseling but are conducted in groups. The workshops or meetings are either fixed (e.g., two hours a week for ten weeks) or open (e.g., meetings every week for two hours without a set ending date). This type of treatment gives parents an opportunity to see that they are not the only ones having problems with their child. It also affords them a chance to discuss their feelings and frustrations with other parents experiencing similar difficulties. Parental workshops and meetings are beneficial to all parents of overactive children.

COUNSELING OR PSYCHOTHERAPY
FOR THE CHILD

There are three general types of counseling or psychotherapy—group, family, and individual.

Group Therapy
Group therapy involves the child meeting with one or two therapists and several other children (usually three to seven) of the same ages experiencing similar difficulties. This type of treatment may include discussions, play, activities, or a combination of these. The goals may be socialization (i.e., helping the child deal more effectively with his or her peers), educational information (e.g.,

how to express anger, what to do if someone teases you), dealing with underlying feelings, building confidence, and so on.

Family Therapy
Family therapy is similar to group therapy, but the "group" involves the child and his or her family members, as well as the therapist. In this situation problems with interaction and communication within the family unit are treated.

Individual Therapy
With individual counseling or psychotherapy, the child meets with a therapist. As in group therapy this may involve discussion, play, and activities. The goals may be similar to those above and are usually based on the child's individual needs and problems.

Individual and group counseling or psychotherapy is more beneficial for children whose overactivity is related to emotional problems. However, some forms of group and family therapy may also help children whose overactivity is not related to emotional difficulties.

MAKING THERAPY EFFECTIVE

If your child becomes involved in counseling or psychotherapy, you should have a general understanding of the process and its results. Here are some questions to ask the therapist to give you a better understanding and increase your involvement.

When therapy is recommended or during your initial meeting with the therapist, you could ask

1. What exactly is my child's problem?
2. How will therapy help?
3. What are the goals of therapy?
4. How will the goals be accomplished?
5. How much will I be involved?
6. How long do you expect therapy to last?
7. How much will this cost?

Once the child is in treatment, you should be *regularly* meeting with the therapist to discuss your child's progress and what you can do to help at home. Some questions that may be discussed during these meetings follow.

1. How is my child progressing?
2. What areas still need improvement?
3. What can I be doing at home to help?
4. How do I deal with stubbornness, temper tantrums, et cetera?
5. His teacher says he is fighting in school, not completing his work, and so on. What should I tell her?
6. Is there anything I can read to give me a better understanding of my child and how to deal with her?
7. When can the therapy sessions begin to be spread out and less frequent?

When therapy has ended, you may ask the therapist

1. What are some things I should look for if she starts slipping back?
2. How often should I call to tell you what is happening?
3. How often should I have his teacher report to me or you?

Be sure that the questions you ask are answered in terms you can understand. After the parents' conference be sure you are not more confused. If you do not understand what is being said, assume that it is the therapist's fault and not that you are not smart enough to understand.

All parents of overactive children, regardless of the cause, would benefit from parental counseling in effective techniques of child management. Individual therapy should primarily be employed when the child is experiencing emotional difficulties. Group therapy may be beneficial for all types of overactive children. However, group therapy will only be effective if it is geared toward the child's specific problems (e.g., peer problems, socialization difficulties, building self-confidence). As with group therapy, family therapy may be beneficial for all types of overactive children when there are problems within the family unit.

chapter ten
SCHOOL INTERVENTIONS

Overactive children almost always experience difficulty in school. Their problems are generally related to academic performance, behavior, or a combination of these. Whether a child is having trouble completing his work, passing tests, getting along with other children, following classroom procedure, understanding her work, or any other performance or behavior in the school setting, communication between the parent and teacher or administration is an absolute necessity. Establish an open line of communication between yourself and the appropriate school personnel (e.g., counselor, teacher, principal). By doing this, you can stay on top of the problem and deal with it before it gets out of hand.

ESTABLISHING COMMUNICATION WITH THE SCHOOL

Very frequently I hear parents say, "They didn't tell me she was in danger of failing until the end of the year." "If he has been a behavior problem since September, why didn't I know about it sooner?" or "If we would have known about her not paying attention when it started, we could have done something about it. Now it's out of hand." Or they wait for the first PTA meeting or parent-teacher conference to make their first contact with the school; this might be two to four months into the school year.

Waiting for the first meeting or for the teacher to contact you is a very bad practice, especially if you have a child with a history of difficulty in school or you suspect he or she is overactive. Most of us forget that although we have one child in Ms. Smith's class, she may have 30 to 175 other students. Therefore, her time may be limited. In addition, teachers are frequently negatively reinforced when they call parents—the parents may be uncooperative or disinterested, blame the school or teacher for the problems, or defend the child and not hear what is said.

The majority of teachers are very concerned about their students and like teaching. So when a teacher encounters a cooperative and concerned parent, he or she will usually bend over backward to open the lines of communication. Even in these situations it is usually better if the parents initiate the contact rather than waiting for the teacher to call. Do not assume that "no news is good news." I often suggest that the parents put an X on a calendar every two or three weeks to remind them to make contact with the teacher. Most of the techniques I use to obtain information from the school are designed to require very little of the teacher's time each day or week, usually three to fifteen seconds. Some of these techniques will be discussed below. The reason for attempting to minimize extra work for teachers, principals, or counselors is simple. If they have to write a note or call you and thirty other parents on Friday, it becomes a monumental task. However, checking a chart or form for thirty students that takes three to five seconds each, only requires two to three minutes.

While a significant number of overactive children have difficulty with their schoolwork because of their behavior, some have learning problems. However, before we can say that an overactive child has a learning problem, his or her behavior must be controlled.

DETERMINING THE PROBLEM

Although all children who have behavior problems do not have learning problems, almost all children who have learning difficulties eventually develop behavior problems. A child may start out having only academic trouble, but after a few months or years of not being able to grasp the material, he will not be able to "keep up." Therefore, he will find himself in a situation where he does not understand what is going on. It may be like he is in a foreign country—very little makes sense.

Suppose I made you and a friend come to a workshop that will last six hours and be given in French. You do not understand French. How would you feel and behave? You would probably sit and pay attention for a while but then would start daydreaming. You would think about what you did yesterday and what you are going to do tonight or Saturday. If I continued to make you sit in this boring situation that made very little sense, you would probably start talking to your friend, making your grocery list, getting up and walking around, and you would soon be a behavior problem and look overactive. Children who have trouble learning experience something similar. In addition, they experience a great deal of failure, frustration, and negative attention and eventually are identified as having behavior problems.

The main reason to establish good communication between parent and teacher is to be aware of and deal with school problems early, before they get out of hand. This is extremely important in effectively remedying academic difficulties. The sooner the problem can be identified, diagnosis determined, and appropriate recommendations made, the easier it is to treat the problem and the less probable it is that future behavior and attitude problems will develop. Many times I see children in fifth and sixth grade who have been having academic problems since kindergarten or first grade, but for some reason nothing has been done earlier.

SEEKING PROFESSIONAL EVALUATION

If a child is experiencing problems with schoolwork, I strongly suggest that you seek out a professional evaluation as soon as possible. Most school systems have evaluation teams to test and diagnose children who are experiencing learning difficulties. The evaluator should also make recommendations to minimize the child's difficulties. Evaluations can also be obtained from mental health centers or other state agencies or private psychologists. Or you could ask the child's pediatrician, teacher, or school to recommend somebody. Evaluations are extremely helpful in assisting children with learning or behavior problems in school. In addition to overactivity, children have trouble with schoolwork for numerous other reasons. They may have learning problems relating to perceptual-motor deficits, auditory or visual processing problems, memory, and so on. The child may have a poor foundation, be at an achievement level below her grade placement (i.e., in fifth grade but reading at a third grade level), or be a slow learner. Appropriate testing will help pinpoint the area or areas of difficulty. In addition, always have a child evaluated *before* he or she repeats a grade. Some children may benefit from repeating, but for others special education is necessary to "correct" their learning problems.

CHANGING TOTAL BEHAVIOR PATTERNS

When an overactive child shows both behavior and academic problems, it is necessary to zero in on the behavior before an accurate assessment of the learning problem can be made. For example, if a child is doing poorly but is not completing work or not paying attention in class, we would have to eliminate the interfering behavior before we could say there is a learning problem. Working to develop appropriate behaviors in the school environment is necessary when only this type of problem exists, as well as when the child shows both academic and behavior difficulties.

The biggest mistake most parents make when trying to eliminate behavioral problems in school is to zero in *only* on the school behavior. For example, Joey's major problem is that he does not follow classroom procedure. His parent sets up a beautiful program to deal with this behavior, but it does not work. Why? Mainly because the behavior at school is only part of a large behavioral pattern. If we take a broader look at Joey, we find that his behavior is typical in many other situations. He does not take his bath when told, and he is always late for dinner. At baseball practice he is supposed to throw to second base but usually throws to first base, and so forth. The program fails because the parent is only working with a small portion of the total behavior.

Children who have problems with authority in school usually have similar difficulties at home. The child who forgets his homework, loses her pencil, leaves his coat in the cafeteria usually shows irresponsible behavior at home. A child's behavior is part of the total environment, and to produce change in one area (e.g., school) other situations where the behavior is seen must also be dealt with. If we only isolate 10 percent of the behavior pattern and try to change this, there is a strong probability that our attempts will fail.

Therefore, in working on school behavior problems, I ask the parents to identify situations in the child's *total* environment where this behavior is seen. When first trying to produce change, we focus on the behavior at home and in the neighborhood rather than at school. We "forget" about school. If a child's "not listening" in school is her major difficulty, we try to get her listening at home before we deal with her academic behaviors. If irresponsibility is the main source of trouble, we first try to build responsible actions at home.

There are several reasons for taking this approach. First, we have much more control of the child's behavior at home than at school. Second, in trying to promote change in this fashion, we can deal with a larger portion of the total behavior pattern. That is, the child's overactive behavior in school may only represent 10 percent of the total pattern; in dealing with the behavior at home and in the neighborhood we are actually influencing 90 percent of the pattern. Finally, patterns of behavior developed elsewhere generalize to school. If a child has learned to manipulate her parents to satisfy her needs, get what she wants, and avoid unpleasant situations and duties, there is a strong probability that this behavior will also be seen at school and the child will follow classroom procedure only when she decides to.

Because "bad" behavior developed at home generalizes to school, the reverse process can also occur. By producing change at home, the new or "good" behavior generalizes to school. Often we see the child's behavior improve at school without directly working on it. In attempting to change any behavior, deal with it in the context of the total environment. When it starts to generalize, you will see improvement in areas that you have not directly dealt with.

Once a behavior shows significant improvement at home, the changes generalize to school about two weeks later. However, sometimes this process does not occur easily and something additional needs to be done to help the behavior generalize to school. This is when we start dealing directly with the school behavior. At this time the communication between the parents and the school should be increased.

If the parents have established some control or change at home in the target behavior but a corresponding improvement at school has not occurred, they can place themselves or the control they have established at home in the academic setting by using behavior charts or some similar type of communication. Again, remember that the system should be kept relatively simple and should require a minimal amount of time for the teacher, principal, or counselor. Several of the procedures that I often use are described below, but the number, type, and style of the communication systems that can be used is only limited by the imagination.

SETTING UP A COMMUNICATION SYSTEM

First, the parent and the appropriate school person should meet. At this time the child's behavior should be discussed in great detail—how often it occurs, when, in what situations it is more likely to be seen, exactly what the behavior involves. In other words, the behavior needs to be analyzed to determine the type of system to be employed. After the behavior is discussed, the parent can design the procedure to be used. Once this has been done, the parent and teacher, at separate times, should sit down with the child and explain the system.

TYPES OF COMMUNICATION SYSTEMS

TARGET BEHAVIOR OCCURS
MORE THAN ONCE A DAY

Let's say a child continually talks in class; this is the behavior you are trying to change. Two general types of systems can be set up.

Time Periods
The teacher decides on a logical way to break the day into time periods. Some teachers divide the day according to subjects, others by type of activity, still others use time (e.g., 8:30 to 10:30, 10:30 to lunch). Once this has been established, you construct a chart, usually on a 3" × 5" index card, similar to Chart 10-1.

	Monday	Tuesday	Wednesday	Thursday	Friday
Math					
Science					
Spelling					
English					
Social Studies					

Chart 10.1. Jason's Quiet Chart

The *child* is responsible for bringing the chart to and from school and seeing that the teacher marks it. Next, both the parent and teacher explain the system. "You have been talking a lot in class, so we have set up a chart to help you be quiet. When you do not talk out of turn during a subject [or period of time], the teacher will put a star on that block. If you do talk, you'll get an X in the block." This procedure is followed, and at the end of the day the child brings the chart home and the *parent* then administers a consequence that has already been determined. For example, each star that the child gets during the day may represent five minutes past her bedtime, or the child may be working for a reward at the end of the week.

The teacher either keeps the chart and marks it after each period, or the child keeps it and gives it to the teacher at the appropriate time. Regardless of how the chart is marked, the child is responsible for it, and the parent administers the consequence, not the teacher. When setting up this system, use positive consequences whenever possible. When punishment is used in these situations, the children "forget" to get the charts marked, lose them, and so on to avoid the negative consequence.

Frequency of Behavior

When behaviors occur more than once a day a chart can be set up based on the number of times a day they occur. A chart similar to Chart 10-2 would be constructed.

Let's say the target behavior is completing seat work. You have analyzed the behavior and found that out of the seven things the child has to do during the school day she very seldom com-

<table>
<thead>
<tr><th>Monday</th><th>Tuesday</th><th>Wednesday</th><th>Thursday</th><th>Friday</th></tr>
</thead>
<tbody>
<tr><td>O O
O O
O O
O</td><td>O O
O O
O O
O</td><td>O O
O O
O O
O</td><td>O O
O O
O O
O</td><td>O O
O O
O O
O</td></tr>
</tbody>
</table>

Chart 10.2. Linda's Finishing Work Chart

pletes one. Therefore, you tell her, "I have put seven circles on this chart. For each assignment that you complete, the teacher will put a star over the circle. When you do not finish, you'll get an X. At the end of the day when you bring the chart home, you can trade your stars in for extra play time" or whatever consequence has been determined to be important to the child.

TARGET BEHAVIOR OCCURS ONLY ONCE A DAY

Sometimes the target behavior only occurs or can occur once a day (e.g., refusing to do math).

The child may exhibit one or several different problem behaviors that only occur once a day. For example, Eddie rushes through his math seat work and usually gets it wrong, talks during reading period, and runs to the cafeteria for lunch. To deal with these different behaviors a chart like Chart 10-3 may be set up.

Chart 10.3. Eddie's School Behavior Chart

	Monday	Tuesday	Wednesday	Thursday	Friday
Takes time with Math					
Quiet during Reading					
Walks to Lunch					

It can be brought to and from school less frequently than the others, say once a week.

USING TOKENS

In all of the above examples, tokens could be used instead of charts to communicate information from the school to the parent. A token could be anything the child could transport from school to home—a sticker, a happy face stamped on the child's hand, a poker chip, a piece of a puzzle, a bean or anything else you might think of.

One parent was having trouble with her daugher completing her work in the classroom. The little girl wanted a new doll. The mother bought a bag of marbles and gave it to the teacher. Both the teacher and parent told the girl that every time she completed a sequence of her work she would get a marble to bring home. At home the mother got a jar and put a sign on it that said "Laurie's New Doll." Laurie was told, "Each day you come home from school you put the marbles you have earned in this jar. When it is filled up, we will get your doll." Laurie got the doll in a few weeks.

For younger children the parents could buy stickers and give them to the teacher. A target behavior (e.g., staying in desk) could be identified and then for each time period that the child remained in his desk, he could be given a sticker to be "traded in" for some predetermined consequence.

DEALING WITH SCHOOL
PROBLEMS EFFECTIVELY

1. Do not assume that "no news is good news." The parent should initiate school contacts.

2. Establish an open line of communication between you and the school. You should schedule a meeting with the appropriate school person (i.e., teacher, counselor, or principal) to discuss your child's problem.

3. If behavior problems are a concern, identify situations in the child's total environment (e.g., home and neighborhood) where similar behaviors are seen.

4. At first, focus on changing the behaviors at home and in the neighborhood rather than at school.

5. After some change is seen at home, if the improvement has not generalized to school, focus on the school behaviors.

6. At this point schedule a meeting at school to discuss the child's behavior in detail.

7. At the meeting decide on the type of communication system and how it will be utilized. Design a system that is simple and requires very little of the teacher's time.

8. You should construct or provide the necessary supplies for the communication system.

9. Make the child responsible for getting information to and from school.

10. The teacher should observe the child's behavior and send the appropriate communication home to you.

11. Administer the consequences at home. Use positive consequences (reward) as much as possible.

12. If the system is effectively implemented and the behavior problems do not improve, have the child evaluated so some other specific techniques or management (e.g., medication, counseling) can be considered.

13. If specific learning difficulties are diagnosed, consider special educational services.

SPECIAL EDUCATION

If a child's behavior improves and she still experiences difficulty with her academic work or behavior problems as well as academic troubles continue, she may require some individual instruction or special educational services. The majority of parents have the wrong idea about what special education means; most equate it with mental retardation. When I tell parents, "I think your child will benefit from a resource room or special education class," they often respond, "I thought you just said she was of average intelligence. Why does she need special education?" To view special education as *only* providing services to mentally retarded children is like only looking at the tip of the iceberg.

Special education provides a wide range of services for children who have physical, behavioral, or academic problems or who will benefit from a smaller and more individualized learning environment. Although mentally retarded children are included, they represent only about 10 percent of the children receiving such services. Generally, special education classes are designed for children who are not benefiting from regular class instruction.

TYPES OF SPECIAL EDUCATION

Descriptions of some types of special education classes or resource rooms follow.

Gifted and Talented (G/T)

Gifted and talented classes for children with significantly above average intelligence. Work designed for average students may be below their level and, therefore, some regular classes would be boring for these children. Special education classes individualize work for the child and present it at a stimulating level.

Learning Disabled (LD)

Special education for the learning disabled child is designed for students who have average or above average intelligence but have difficulty learning by regular classroom methods. The special education teacher prescribes work in a manner that will facilitate learning. Children whose overactivity is related to a hyperkinetic reaction of childhood sometimes have learning disabilities. The individual instruction and less frustrating work in special education classes help reduce their overactivity.

Behaviorally or Emotionally Disturbed

This type of special education service is for children who have the ability to learn, but have emotional or behavior problems interfering with their performance in a regular classroom. A small class setting that focuses on behavioral or emotional difficulties is necessary to give these children an opportunity to learn.

Educationally Handicapped

These classes are designed for children who fall within the gray area between average intelligence and mild mental retardation. *Slow learner* means exactly what it says. These children can learn, but at a pace somewhat slower than the child of average intelligence. For example, you are an average student and I am a slow learner. The teacher gives us ten math problems and fifteen minutes to complete them. You finish all ten, but I only complete six. However, give me another ten minutes and I will finish all of them. Therefore, special education classes for slow learners are designed to present work at a rate commensurate to students' learning style. Some children who fall in the lower part of the slow learner range of intelligence may show overactive behaviors. Special educational placement may reduce the difficulty they experience because of their behavior.

Mentally Retarded

This type of special educational service is designed for children whose level of intelligence falls below the slow learner range. It is usually of two types. Classes for the mildly mentally retarded are designed for children who can learn but only to a certain level. Classes for the moderately mentally retarded are designed to teach children personal self-sufficiency and how to get along in society. Some retarded children show overactive behaviors, and special class placement will help alleviate these.

Physically Handicapped

A variety of special education services are available for children with physical difficulties that interfere with their ability to perform in a regular class. This may include children who are orthopedically handicapped (e.g., cerebral palsy), are sight or hearing impaired, or have speech difficulties. Classes are designed to meet the physical needs of the child, provide the necessary remediation (such as speech therapy), and have learning materials designed to compensate for the physical impairment (e.g., special materials designed for children in wheelchairs or with sight or hearing deficits).

Multiply Handicapped

These special education classes are designed to provide services for children experiencing a combination of the difficulties described above.

SPECIAL EDUCATION CLASSES

Special education is designed to meet the educational needs of a variety of students who would have difficulty with or would not benefit from a regular classroom setting. These students would not learn by the methods employed to teach the majority of students.

There are generally two types of special education classes—self-contained classes and resource rooms. In a self-contained special education class, the child usually remains in the same classroom and receives specialized services for the entire day. The resource room provides children with part-time services in deficient areas. The child attends regular classes for part of the day, and the other part receives individual attention in weak subjects in a special education class. Resource rooms are more common in public school settings and are used in an attempt to avoid labeling and to have the child in as many "regular" classes as he or she can handle.

The advantages of special education are twofold. First, it allows a smaller pupil-teacher ratio than regular classes. By having fewer students the teacher can give more individual attention and can present the work in a manner or at a rate commensurate with the child's strengths and weaknesses. The special education teacher can utilize the child's strong areas to build his or her weak areas.

The second goal of special education is to make learning a pleasant and positive experience to keep the child motivated. Many children who require special education have had months, if not years, of failure, frustration, and negative attention in the academic environment. Because they cannot compete in a regular classroom and their weaknesses have been continually emphasized, they "turn off" to school and lack interest in or concern for academic work. They may avoid sitting down in front of a book or doing anything that resembles schoolwork. Special education classes are designed to present work in a fashion that will assure success and achievement. This, combined with teacher emphasis on the child's accomplishments and strong points, maintains the child's interest and motivation in academic endeavors.

It is estimated that about one out of every ten students needs some form of special educational service. Some children will experience monumental difficulties in school if they do not receive this type of help. Therefore, special education is a very important aspect of our school systems, and parents should be willing to take advantage of its services.

Special education is primarily designed for children who are experiencing learning difficulties. While some overactive children will fall into one of the above categories, a large portion of them will not. Many overactive children's problems in school are related to the characteristics of overactivity, specifically behavioral or adjustment difficulties. If the overactive child does not fit into one of the above classifications, special class placement cannot be made, and his or her school behavior must be dealt with by one of the methods discussed earlier.

chapter eleven

DIET AND NUTRITION

During the past fifty years reports have linked overactivity to food allergies. In recent years, there has been much study of dietary or nutritional management of overactive behaviors in children. This technique is primarily related to hyperactivity. The two major theorists in this area are Ben Feingold and Lendon Smith.

THE FEINGOLD DIET

I will not attempt to discuss the Feingold Diet in great detail, but will try to give you a general idea of what is involved. I strongly suggest that the interested reader obtain the *Feingold Cookbook For Hyperactive Children*, as well as Dr. Feingold's other book, *Why Your Child Is Hyperactive*, both published by Random House, for further details.

In the Feingold Diet two groups of foods are eliminated. Group I foods contain natural salicylates and include fruits and vegetables. The list of these fruits and vegetables, which must be omitted from the child's diet in all forms—fresh, frozen, canned, dried, as juice or as ingredients of prepared foods—follows.

Almonds	Nectarines
Apples	Oranges
Apricots	Peaches

Blackberries	Pickles
Boysenberries	Plums
Cherries	Prunes
Cucumbers	Raisins
Currants	Raspberries
Gooseberries	Strawberries
Grapes	Tomatoes

Group II is made up of all foods that contain synthetic (artificial) color or flavor. This diet is *not* concerned with food preservatives, except butylated hydroxytoluene (BHT) to which some children may show an adverse response. But all foods that contain artificial color and flavors must be eliminated from the child's diet. To determine if a product contains artificial coloring or flavoring, you must read the label carefully.

The following is a general list of items that are *not* permitted on the Feingold Diet. It will give you a feel for some of the foods that must be avoided.

All cereals with artificial colors and flavors

All instant-breakfast preparations

All manufactured cakes, cookies, pastries, sweet rolls, doughnuts, pie crusts, or other bakery products

Frozen baked goods and many packaged baking mixes

Bologna, salami, frankfurters, meat loaf, or any other artificially flavored or colored luncheon meats

Artificially flavored or colored sausage, ham, bacon, or pork

All barbecued poultry and "self-basting" turkeys

Frozen fish fillets or fish sticks that are dyed or flavored

All manufactured ice cream, sherbet, ices, gelatins, and puddings, except when the label specifies no synthetic coloring or flavoring

All powdered puddings, dessert mixes, and flavored yogurt

All manufactured candies, hard or soft

Diet drinks, soft drinks, cider, all instant-breakfast drinks, all quick-mix powdered drinks, hot or cold tea, and prepared chocolate milk

Oleomargarine, colored butter, mustard, catsup, colored cheeses, wine or cider vinegar, commercial chocolate syrup, cloves, chili sauce, and all mint-flavored items

Medications and vitamins containing artificial flavors or colors, as well as over-the-counter medications that contain aspirin (e.g., Anacin, Alka-Seltzer, Bufferin, Excedrin)

> All toothpastes, toothpowder, mouthwashes, cough drops, throat lozenges, and antacid tablets

As you see, Group II foods comprise the majority of foods eaten by most children. Therefore, grocery shopping must be done carefully, and a number of foods must be homemade. Dr. Feingold also provides a list of foods permitted on the diet. A summary of this list follows.

> All meats, fresh fish, and poultry (except stuffed)
> All commercial breads except egg and whole wheat (usually dyed)
> Any dry or cooked cereal without artificial colors or flavors
> Tapioca, plain yogurt, natural (white) cheese, and honey
> Distilled white vinegar, all cooking oils and fats, and all flours
> Grapefruit and pineapple juice, pear and guava nectar, Seven-Up, and milk
> Homemade items made *without* artificial colors, flavors, or the foods listed in Group I. A partial list follows:

bakery items	james or jellies
candies	lemonade
chocolate syrup	limeade
custards	mayonnaise
gelatins	mustard
ice cream	puddings

> All other foods that do not contain natural salicylates (Group I) or artificial flavors or colors (Group II)

If a child shows a favorable response to the Feingold Diet after four to six weeks, the foods in Group I may be slowly restored. New foods from Group I must be introduced one at a time. They should be tried for three or four days, and if no unfavorable reaction in the child's behavior is noted, another food item can be added. This procedure is followed until all items in Group I are tested. Those fruits and vegetables to which the child does not show an adverse reaction can be included in the diet. For example, a child who shows a favorable response to the diet may be given a trial on tomatoes or tomato gravy. If he does not show an increased level of activity or attentional problems when eating this food, it can be included in his diet. However, if the child shows an adverse reaction, the food should be discontinued. Regardless of the child's reaction, another item from Group I can be introduced after a period of time.

Dr. Feingold offers some general instructions for parents who have children on his diet. Some of these follow.

1. A diet diary must be kept. Everything the child eats must be noted. In addition, it is usually helpful to record the child's behavioral and academic responses. Whenever a change in behavior occurs, suspect a diet infraction.

2. The probability of success and eliminating resistance from the child is greatly increased if the whole family goes on the diet.

3. There must be strict adherence to the diet, 100 percent. It is all or none. There cannot be any cheating.

4. No restrictions are placed on homemade quantities of sweets.

5. All package and container labels should be read carefully. When in doubt, do not use them.

6. If improvement occurs, it will be observed on the average within one to three weeks. For some children improvement may not be seen until seven weeks.

7. In some cases drugs used to control hyperactive behaviors can be discontinued after the child has been on the diet for two or three weeks. However, the child's doctor should always be contacted before the medication is changed or reduced.

DR. SMITH'S NUTRITIONAL APPROACH

Dr. Lendon Smith feels that everyone should follow a general eating pattern as part of a lifetime program of good nutrition. He calls this pattern of eating the Prevention Diet. In addition to this general diet, he makes specific recommendations to control the symptoms of overactivity. For more information on his ideas, see Dr. Smith's books, *Feed Your Kids Right*, and *Improving Your Child's Behavior Chemistry*, Prentice-Hall, Inc., 1976.

The Prevention Diet has three parts.

1. Antinutrients should be avoided. This generally involves foods that have been packaged, processed, added to, stabilized,

emulsified, colored, or preserved. In general, commercial products should be avoided as much as possible. Sugar and "junk" foods are not permitted. Some of the foods that have to be eliminated are

white and brown sugar	commercial ice cream
corn, cane, or maple syrup	boxed cereal
molasses	white flour
honey	homogenized, pasteurized milk for a month

2. Natural foods should be eaten four to six times a day, in small amounts. Some of these follow.

raw vegetables	fish
eggs	chicken
white cheeses (jack, Swiss, mozzarella)	vegetables (such as peas, beans, and lentils)
nuts (especially almonds and peanuts)	raw fruits

3. Begin daily vitamins and minerals (assuming the child is behind in the requirements).

Vitamins

A: 5,000–10,000 units

B complex: 25–50 mg (Should contain 25 mg each of B_1, B_2 B_3 (niacinamide), B_6 (pyridoxine), Inositol, Choline, PABA, pantothenic acid; 25 mcg of B_{12}, 250 mcg of biotin, 400 mcg of folic acid.)

Minerals

Calcium: 500–1,000 mg

Copper: 1.0 mg

Iodine: 0.1 mg

Magnesium: 250–500 mg

Manganese: 5 mg

Zinc: 5 mg

In addition to the Prevention Diet, Dr. Smith gives some suggestions to deal with symptoms of overactivity.

Hyperactivity

Dr. Smith states that some behaviors characterized as hyperactive can be managed by the following procedure called the Stress Formula.

1. Eat no sugar, white flour, packaged cereals or the like
2. Nibble nutritious foods every two to three hours
3. Take vitamin C, 500–10,000 mg per day
4. Take vitamin B complex, 50–200 mg of each of the Bs per day for a month or so, then a lower dose, perhaps, for life
5. Take pantothenic acid 500–3,000 mg per day. This can be varied up or down
6. Take pyridoxine (B_6) in doses of 200–500 mg per day
7. Take vitamin A, 30,000–50,000 units per day for a month
8. Take calcium, as dolomite or bone meal or a calcium salt, in doses up to 1,000 mg per day

Dr. Smith also states that some overactivity in children may be reduced by B complex vitamin injections. B_6 in 200–500 mg doses may help. Often, large doses of calcium (1,000–2,000 mg per day) plus vitamin D (500–1,000 units per day) will result in improvement. Extra zinc (50–90 mg per day) may be a partial answer.

Short Attention Span

To reduce a child's distractibility, attentional problems, and concentration deficits, Smith recommends:

1. Exclude salicylates (see Feingold Diet) and food additives
2. Increase B complex vitamins to 100–200 mg of each
3. Increase nutritious foods
4. Increase calcium and magnesium

Clumsiness

An increase in B complex vitamins, especially B_6 (100 mg per day), may improve a child's coordination.

In a recent letter briefly explaining how his nutritional approach can be used to manage overactive behaviors, Dr. Smith wrote,

In general I have found that if a child is hyperactive, as defined by whatever criteria the teacher may use, I can help that child achieve to the maximum of his potential if he/she has the following: ticklishness, Jekyll and Hyde behavior, food and carbohydrate cravings, deep or light sleep habits, bed-wetting, and some rhythmical tension-relieving activity (thumb sucking, rocking, nail biting). The above findings indicate to me that the child does have a biochemical problem and [it] can be solved with a nutritional approach. Mainly: no sugar, white flour, boxed cereals, junk, additives, and all dairy products. [He or she is] to nibble on good wholesome foods and take extra vitamins and minerals, specifically vitamins C, B complex (especially B_6), and calcium and magnesium. Eighty percent will be 60 percent to 100 percent better in three weeks if I use the above criteria (7,000 cases now). Another fairly reliable test: If Ritalin or Dexedrine have a calming effect then I know that the patient has a biochemical defect and a nutritional approach will help. I can usually guarantee that the dose of medication can be reduced or eliminated in three weeks.

In another correspondence Dr. Smith wrote,

I use the B complex shots on all of the children that I can get a hold of. The B_6 vitamin seems to be the most important one of the Bs. Apparently these children have an absorption problem, and the shots are almost a necessity once or twice a week for three weeks to get things going. I am amazed at how commonly these children have allergies that somehow hurt the intestinal tract so that they are unable to absorb the calcium and maybe the B vitamins. We do hair tests on these children and find that they are almost universally low in calcium and magnesium. It appears that they do not absorb the calcium from milk. Many hyper children crave milk or sugar or the very food that is causing their disagreeable behavior.

EFFECTIVENESS OF DIET AND NUTRITIONAL PROGRAMS

Although there does seem to be some relationship between what a child eats and his or her level of activity, research is somewhat limited. It seems that a child's body chemistry as it combines with certain food additives is highly individual. That is, eliminating certain chemicals from the diet or having a child eat certain foods may work for him, but not for another child. I have had some parents tell me that a diet produced significant improvement in their child's activity level. However, it seems that for every parent who has reported positive results, a large number have told me that diet did not improve their child's overactivity.

Several things must be kept in mind when considering dietary methods.

- Diets that eliminate certain flavor or color additive chemicals in food or provide nutritious foods seem to work on an individual basis and result in positive improvement for some children, but not for all.
- If a parent decides to use this method of treatment, there must be strict adherence to the diet. It is all or none. There cannot be any "cheating."
- The probability of success and eliminating resistance from the child is greatly increased if the whole family goes on the diet. It is very difficult to tell a child he cannot drink a Coke if his sister is drinking one.
- The diets are somewhat difficult to follow because most prepared foods and many fresh fruits and vegetables must be eliminated. Since the meals prepared often must be made from scratch and utilize natural or raw foods, they may involve more time and be viewed as "troublesome."

The dietary and nutritional management of overactive behaviors in children is a relatively new concept, but has received a great deal of attention in recent years. I have not seen enough research or positive results to make me a firm believer in this method of management. However, I do not like to see children on medication and usually try to exhaust every other alternative before I recommend drugs to control the interfering symptoms of overactivity. Therefore, when parents ask me about diet I give them general information along wtih the pluses and minuses. I also recommend that they purchase Dr. Feingold's and/or Dr. Smith's book(s) to get more detailed information. I feel that anything is worth a try to avoid having a child on medication. It may work, and we may be able to avoid drugs.

chapter twelve

MEDICATION

Medication is one way to deal with overactive behavior, but most parents and professionals do not like to use it before other things are tried. These are my feelings exactly. If the techniques outlined in Part II are successfully implemented and overactive behaviors continue, then some of the specific techniques outlined in Part III can be tried. If all the nondrug methods to deal with the behavior are adequately employed and are unsuccessful, it becomes appropriate to consider medication.

Only after an effective behavior management program has been initiated in the home or other environment interventions are made and the child continues to show overactive behavior should medication be tried. Medication should always be used in conjunction with counseling for parents in effective techniques of child management. Different drugs are used to treat different types of overactivity.

HYPERACTIVITY: HYPERKINETIC REACTION OF CHILDHOOD (ATTENTIONAL DEFICIT DISORDER)

In this type of overactivity, which results from a developmental lag or deviation, the child does not have sufficient control to prevent his behavior or enable him to sit still or concentrate for long periods of time.

Central nervous system stimulants, such as Ritalin, Dexedrine, or Cylert, are most often used to manage hyperactivity. Some medication has the opposite from the expected effect in hyperactive children. For example, the above medications are stimulants. If you or I took them, they would speed us up and make us overactive. However, these medications appear to "slow down" a hyperactive child. On the other hand, if you give a hyperactive child a tranquilizer or drug that would slow us down or put us to sleep, it usually increases her activity level and she stays up all night.

The medications used with children diagnosed as hyperkinetic are central nervous system stimulants, which activate certain parts of the body. The central nervous system is the basis for a child's control. Therefore, the medication stimulates it to give the child more control. In general, the child is easier to manage and shows fewer school-related problems. The medication (the shaded area in Figure 12-1) indirectly benefits the child by giving him more controls. He is not sedated or "doped up." In other words, his controls catch up with his "motor."

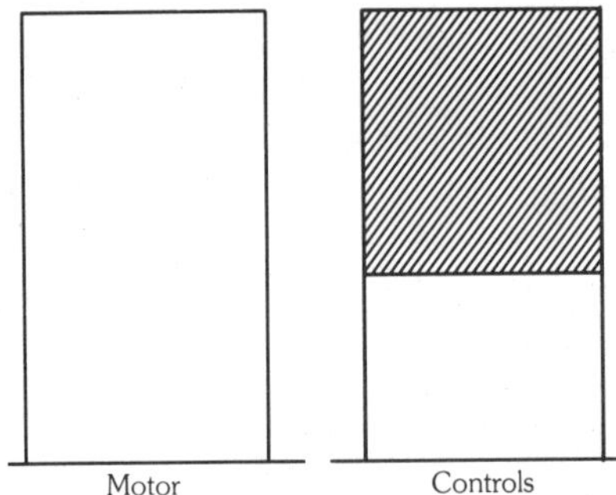

Figure 12.1. Effect of Medication on Hyperactive Child's Controls Related to "Motor"

The medication helps control the interfering symptoms of hyperactivity. Not only does it help the child sit still and fidget less, but it also improves span of attention and decreases distractibility.

Hyperactive children usually experience great difficulty in the classroom. Cognitive overactivity (e.g., short attention span, inability to concentrate, distractibility) poses the greatest obstacle to their school performance.

Suppose I start to give you directions on how to get to my house. However, there are seven people behind me—one is telling funny stories, one is giving the weather, one is telling jokes, and so on. As I start giving directions—"You go down Judge Perez Drive until you get to the second red light"—you hear a good joke and start paying attention to the "joke man." Then, while you are listening to him, you catch some interesting bit of weather and you start concentrating on the "weather woman." As I continue talking, you are repeatedly distracted by one of the people standing behind me. Now, you focus your attention back to me and hear, "It's the the third house from the corner." I ask, "Do you know how to get to my house?" and your answer would be "No." Your negative answer is not because you do not understand my directions or because you are not smart. The reason you cannot answer the question is that you did not receive the information—you were distracted or you did not concentrate on what I was saying.

This is often what happens to a hyperactive child in the classroom. His performance is poor because he is easily distracted or cannot attend to the teacher for a long period of time and, therefore, he never receives the information. Consequently, when he is tested or has to perform, he fails. The medication does not make a child smarter or able to learn faster, but it does eliminate the interfering symptoms of hyperactivity. In the above example, it would eliminate the seven people standing behind me. Now you would be able to attend to my directions and find my house, provided you were capable of understanding the directions.

RESULTS OF HYPERACTIVITY MEDICATION

If you give any child one of the medications mentioned earlier, one of four things will happen.

1. The medication will "calm her down." She will be less active and more able to concentrate for longer periods of time. She will be able to control herself better, the majority of her "hyperactive" symptoms will decrease, and she generally will show a positive improvement. If this occurs, you know she is hyperactive and the dose is adequate.

2. Nothing happens. The child does not show any significant

change. If this occurs, the child may be hyperactive but not be receiving enough medication.

3. The child may appear drowsy, as if she is tired, and may fall asleep when looking at TV or when she sits still. When this occurs, she probably is hyperactive but receiving too much medication.

4. The child may become more active. If this occurs, the child is not hyperactive, and the medication should be discontinued.

You should *not* increase or decrease the dosage of your child's medication without consulting your child's doctor. Therefore, if reactions 2 through 4 occur, contact your child's doctor. You can usually see one of the above results in one to seven days after the child starts taking the medication. Most physicians start with the minimal amount of medication. The effects are then observed, and if there are no positive results the amount of medication is increased. During the time you are first giving the child medication, it is very important to keep in touch with your child's doctor. Because most medication is given for school problems and is primarily given during the school hours (i.e., before breakfast and before lunch), it is necessary to get reports from the child's teacher. The teacher should be informed when the child starts the medication and should be asked to report immediately any behavioral changes.

QUESTIONS ABOUT HYPERACTIVITY MEDICATION

Most parents who give children medication for hyperactivity have many questions regarding the drugs and their effects. Here are some of the typical questions asked by parents, along with brief answers.

Is there a risk of drug dependency in later years? No. Years of clinical experience and research have failed to reveal an association between the medical use of stimulants in the young child and later drug abuse. Physicians who care for children treated with stimulants observe that most often they are willing to stop the therapy, which they view as "medicine." Therefore, the young child's experience of drug effects under medical management does not seem to induce misuse.

How long will the child have to take the medication? This is a difficult question to answer specifically because it is different for every child. However, most children take the medication until they reach puberty, somewhere between the ages of eleven and sixteen. Because this type of overactivity is a result of developmental lags and the child is growing daily, the gap between "motor" and controls is constantly changing. Therefore, there is some possibility, although minimal, that the child will "outgrow" the hyperactivity before puberty. Most of the pediatricians I work with tend to take the child off the medication at the start of school and right after the Christmas holidays to see if the child has developed additional controls and if the medication is still necessary.

What if the medication does not work and appears to have little or no effect on the child's behavior? Consult your child's doctor. There is a possibility that she is hyperactive but needs a stronger dose of the same medication. Or your child may require a different type of medication.

What should I do if the child has to take other medication for a sore throat, cold, allergy, or other illness? Consult your child's doctor. Some medications can be taken with other drugs, some cannot.

Will the child be "doped up"? What does the medication do? No, the child will not be "doped up." The medication seems to activate a part of the child's body and give him more controls. Therefore, the medication seems indirectly to "calm down" a child.

If I am giving the child the medication to improve school behavior and performance, do I have to give it on weekends, holidays, and during the summer? Consult your child's doctor. Some physicians require the child to take the medication all the time; others suggest that the child be on the medication only when in school.

How long do the effects of the medication last? For Ritalin and Dexedrine, the effects usually wear off in three to four hours. A child taking these drugs usually takes a dose in the morning and a dose at lunchtime to cover the entire school day. If the child's overactive behavior is a concern at home, the child may also take another dose when he comes home from school.

Cylert's effects are longer lasting, about six hours, and a child on this medication usually receives only one dose in the morning.

What is a minimal dose of medication? This is different for different children and usually depends on the child's size. However, most physicians prescribing Ritalin or Dexedrine start the child on 5–10 mg twice a day. With Cylert the dosage is 18.75 to 37.50 mg once a day. If needed, this is gradually increased.

Are there any side effects with these medications? Loss of appetite and inability to fall asleep are the most common side effects. These can be reduced by giving the child the medication before meals and no later than 3:00 P.M. However, most children become tolerant to these side effects within the first week or two of treatment.

Other side effects, which occur less frequently, include mild stomach aches and headaches and increased "tension" behaviors, including nail biting, eye blinking, sensitivity, or moodiness. When these occur the type of medication may have to be changed. If side effects continue, contact your child's doctor.

The above are the short-term effects of the drugs used with hyperactive children. There is little research evidence of the long-term risks of stimulant medication. There are suggestions of a period of growth suppression. However, over a longer period of time, the loss of expected growth is made up.

When will I know if the medication is working? Sometimes you can tell within a few hours of giving the child the medication. However, it may take a week to see the effects of Ritalin and Dexedrine. Improvement may not be evident until the third or fourth week with Cylert.

What will happen if the child needs the medication, but I decide not to give it to her? There is little hard data on the long-term adverse physical effects of the medication. However, we know the long-term detrimental psychological and educational effects in hyperactive children who do not receive medication. Usually a hyperactive child not on medication will receive a great deal of negative attention and correction. Consequently, there is a strong possibility that he or she will develop a negative self-image. In addition, although they may be bright, the interfering symptoms of hyperactivity prevent children from learning, and they fall further and further behind in school.

Does the medication interfere with healthy psychological development or handicap the child emotionally? No. For the hyperactive child the medication gives more controls, reduces the negative attention he or she will receive, and enhances satisfactory psychological development.

SIGNIFICANT EMOTIONAL DIFFICULTIES

Children whose overactivity is resulting from emotional difficulties sometimes respond to stimulant drugs. Because these drugs are usually safer than those used for emotional difficulties, the children are often first given a trial on a stimulant, even though it will probably not decrease the level of activity. The most commonly used drugs for overactivity resulting from emotional problems are Thorazine, Mellaril, Stelazine, or similar drugs. These medications are usually prescribed by a psychiatrist and should be given in conjunction with some type of psychotherapy.

INTELLIGENCE

Children who have a depressed level of intelligence often show symptoms of overactivity. These children's symptoms usually result from brain damage. Sometimes stimulants work with these children. Those used for children with emotional problems seem to be most effective. However, medication often does not seem to reduce the overactivity resulting from this cause. Therefore, the parents must set up a very structured environment and may have to tolerate some overactive behaviors in this type of child.

Children whose overactive behavior relates to high levels of intelligence are generally not managed by medication, although sometimes the stimulant medications are used. Effective management techniques must be employed, and parents of this type of child may have to tolerate some overactive behaviors.

MANAGEMENT

Medication is not used with children whose overactive behavior results from a lack of or ineffective management technique, personality characteristics, attitude, or learned behavior patterns.

COMBINED CAUSES

When overactivity results from a combination of factors, medication may be employed. However, other techniques are first tried to reduce the overactivity before drugs are used.

IV
PROBLEMS COMMON TO OVERACTIVE CHILDREN

chapter thirteen

ATTITUDE AND BEHAVIOR CHARACTERISTICS

SHORT ATTENTION SPAN

Most overactive children show deficits in the areas of attention and concentration. They are described as "easily distracted," "unable to concentrate for more than a short period of time," "daydreamers." Often, it may be difficult to eliminate problems in this area totally, but several things can be done to improve the child's ability to concentrate, as well as to reduce the hassle that may be produced by this weakness.

Reduce Distractions

If the child who is easily distracted attempts to do his homework in the kitchen, where his mother is cooking, his sister is also doing her homework, and his baby brother is playing on the floor, he is certain to experience problems. Many things are happening that will easily take his attention away from his homework. Consequently, it may appear that he is never going to finish.

Imagine yourself at a party where seven different and interesting people are talking at one time. You are in the middle and listening to Person 1, but Person 4 says something that gets your attention. Then Person 6 starts telling an amusing story, so you begin listening to him, and so forth. After an hour you may be totally confused, not fully understand what anyone is talking about, and if you were trying to perform some task you would not have finished. This is exactly how an overactive child feels when he or she is bombarded with stimuli or is in a situation that involves many distractions.

When trying to get a child who has attentional problems to perform a task (e.g., homework), he should be placed in an environment with minimal distraction. He should *not* be in a room where other activity is going on, a TV is running, or people or things can divert his attention from the task. Place him in a quiet room, a part of the house that does not have much "people traffic." Reduce both distractions that can be heard (e.g., voices of children playing outside, sound of TV) and seen (e.g., activity outside a window, favorite toys).

Break Up Tasks into Small Units

Suppose a child has fifteen minutes of homework that drag into hours primarily because she can only concentrate for short periods of time. It may not be wise to try to get her to do it all at one time. You could break it up into three five-minute sessions. The length of the sessions will vary for each child. For some children I have started off using thirty-second or one-minute time periods. For example, you may tell a child, "We are going to break up your homework. We'll do some now and then some later."

For some children positive consequences will also help improve their ability to concentrate. In the above example you would tell the child the same thing but add, "I'm going to set the timer on the stove for five minutes, and if you work the whole time till the bell rings, I will play that game you like to play." As the child improves, or if small periods of time are at first used, the length of the sessions can be increased. For example, you may start off with one-minute sessions for several days. When the child is doing well, the time periods could be increased to two minutes. This could be done until you reach the maximum time that the child can concentrate at one sitting.

In addition to breaking up the task into time periods, the task itself can be broken up. Suppose a child's room has been messed up for days and you tell him, "Go clean up your room." The child goes in the room and starts picking up, but after he has made his bed and put his shoes away, he finds a toy that has been lost for weeks. Naturally, he stops what he is doing and starts playing. Fifteen minutes later you find that the room is still a mess. The task of cleaning the room may involve several separate duties (e.g., making a bed, putting away toys, hanging up clothes, picking up shoes, putting dirty clothes where they belong), and overactive children who have attentional problems usually have trouble with this type of situation.

To make this task easier, decrease the hassle involved, and increase the probability of success, the child could be given the duties involved in getting a room clean one at a time. For example, he could be told, "Go make your bed." After a period of time he would be told, "Go hang up your clothes," and so forth. Consequences could also be used in this situation (e.g., "You cannot go play until your bed is made," "I'll play pitch and catch with you when all your clothes are hung up"). The number of duties that the child is required to do at one time can be increased as he improves. However, you may never get to the point where you can tell him, "Go clean your room."

Give Instructions One at a Time

A child with attentional problems is told, "Go outside and take this food to the dog. When you are outside bring in the mop and tell your brother to come inside." She goes outside and while putting the food down for the dog to eat, she spots a bug crawling on the side of the house. She starts following it, and five minutes later she comes inside without the mop or her brother. You then ask, "Where's the mop? Did you tell your brother to come inside?" The child responds with "I forgot."

Overactive children with problems in this area cannot handle a series of directions. They may finish the first, but forget about the other two. Usually something distracts the child before she is able to get to the second task and she "forgets" about it. Have her repeat the instructions back to you in her own words.

When giving overactive children directions, be sure they hear and understand what is being said. Often the reason directions are not completed is that they are never heard or fully understood. Because of attentional problems, the child may not be listening to what the parent says. Therefore, be sure you have the child's attention before you give instructions. Look him in the face and have him look at you.

INCREASED ACTIVITY LEVEL

Some of the constant movement, excessive energy, and inability to keep still seen in overactive children may have to be tolerated by their parents. But some can be changed and procedures can be employed that will reduce the hassle, conflict, and negative attention that centers on these behaviors.

One procedure is to rank the overactive behaviors in order of importance or severity. That is, list the child's overactive behaviors from those that could not be tolerated to those that are not so bad. Behaviors at the bottom of the list could be overlooked or tolerated and more attention given to the behaviors at the top of the list. For example, you may not be able to overlook a child's running through the house, but you may be able to tolerate his squirming and fidgetiness while looking at TV.

Allowing the overactive child to participate in physical play and games, to perform house chores, and generally to engage in activities that will "burn up" energy may also help reduce her activity level when she is in the house. However, try to give the child a cooling off period or a time to unwind before she comes inside. Keeping an overactive child "busy" and channeling his activity into some specific task may also help.

Some minor overactivity can be overlooked, but I am not saying that you have to be tolerant of all the child's overactive behaviors. Other behaviors can be modified or reduced. Several procedures that can be employed to accomplish this follow.

Behavior charts can be used with these types of behaviors, because they often occur frequently during the day (see Chapter 7).

A system of warnings and rewards might also be effective. Let's say a child does not sit still during mealtime. He taps his fork, gets up from the table several times, fidgets, and squirms. Mealtime is a hassle and usually results in indigestion for the parents. To decrease the child's activity level at the dinner table, the parents would first identify a reward. They would tell the child, "We are going to give you warnings while we are eating every time you fidget, get up, and so on [explain exactly what the child must do to get the warning]. If you get less than three warnings, we will go get an ice cream after we eat [or whatever the identified reward is]. If you get three or more warnings, we will not get the ice cream." For some children more warnings may have to be used, for others fewer.

Another child may not be able to play quietly. She is constantly making noise, jumping, and running. You would like to decrease her inappropriate activity while playing. You might tell her "If you can play quietly [explain exactly what you mean by this] for a few minutes, we will then play that game you like so much. If you run around and make a lot of noise, we will not play the game." At first, the time the child would have to play quietly would be very short. As she becomes successful and is able to play quietly for the given period, the time could be increased.

These are general ways you can deal with your child's increased levels of activity. Review Part II for additional ideas on how to reduce overactive behaviors.

IMPULSIVENESS

Many overactive children are described as impulsive, not thinking before they act, having poor judgment or foresight. Their parents often state that they show daredevil behavior, a lack of concern for what will happen to them, and a reckless and careless approach to the environment. Although they may have been told many times not to do something and "know" they will be punished, they do it anyway. These behaviors often result in accidents, inappropriate actions, and repeated disciplining.

Reducing impulsive behaviors and getting a child to think before she acts is not an easy task. Generally you have to help the child think about what will happen before she does something or teach the child to weigh the consequences of his behavior before he acts.

Parents can reduce this type of behavior in two general ways. Let's take an example of a child who is continually jumping off a very high porch onto cement. This is dangerous. The child may get hurt, but it appears that he does not care or is not thinking about what will happen to him. One way to deal with this is to talk to the child. Explain what could happen to him and how he could get hurt in an attempt to get him thinking. You should not avoid explaining things to your children. However, do not expect talk to control and reduce this type of behavior. Change is related more to what you do than what you say.

The second and more effective method of reducing this type of behavior is to spell out the rule—"Do not jump off the porch"—and specify a consequence—"If you jump off the porch again, you will have to go sit inside for ten minutes." Whatever happens to the child is then a result of the child's behavior, and he knows about it ahead of time. If this is done consistently over and over again, the child's impulsiveness should start decreasing, and he should begin to think before he acts (see Chapter 3).

The above primarily relates to discipline, but you can also use this method on other behaviors to get a child to think before he or she acts. Not only do you spell out disciplinary measures ahead of time but, for some children, you tie all consequences to their behavior at first.

An example will make this point. Suppose a family is sitting watching TV and the mother all of a sudden tells the child, "Let's go get an ice cream." They get an ice cream and the child enjoys it. However, who is responsible for the pleasure he is experiencing? His mother, because she decided to take him. When trying to get a child to think of the consequences of his behavior before he acts, you would try to relate everything to his behavior. In the above example you may pick something for the child to do before getting the ice cream. It could be something important—"If you go clean your room, we'll get an ice cream, but if your room is not cleaned we will stay home." Or, it could be something relatively unimportant—"If you go get the papers on the bed and bring them to me, we will go get an ice cream, but if you do not we will not go." Regardless of how it is set up, the child earns the ice cream, and he is responsible for the pleasure and enjoyment he experiences. This may enable him to weigh the consequences before he acts.

When trying to establish responsible behaviors in children, it is important to prevent things from "falling out of the sky." The punishment or reward must be directly tied to the child's behavior, and the rules and consequences must be spelled out ahead of time. Playing games or engaging in activities that require planning and foresight may also help. For example, working mazes, model building, playing checkers, sewing, or cooking.

EXCITABILITY AND MOODINESS

Parents of overactive children often describe them as being easily excited, unpredictable, (e.g., calm one minute, excited the next, or sweet and then mean), having poor emotional control, and so forth.

As mentioned earlier in the book, overactive children become more excited and active in unpredictable, fluid, and changing environments. These children are less likely to show these behavioral problems in a structured situation. Therefore, one way to reduce the appearance of these overactive characteristics is to reduce change, uncertainty, and ambiguity in the child's surroundings (see Chapter 3).

Avoid inconsistency—say what you mean and mean what you say. Do not say anything you cannot or do not want to do, and follow through with everything you say. Establish routines in the environment (e.g., set bedtime, bath time). Avoid "maybes" and "ifs," statements like "If I can get off work early tomorrow, I'll come home and we'll play baseball." "Maybe we'll go to Grandma's tomorrow if she is home." Deal in certainties. Do not tell the child about something unless you know it is going to happen.

This brings me to another important point—when do you tell an overactive child about an event? Although you want to make the environment predictable and not do things on the spur of the moment, if you tell an excitable child about an event too far in advance, he is apt to drive you crazy with questions. You have to reach a happy medium. Let's say a child is to go to a birthday party Saturday at 3:00 P.M. If her parent tells her this at 9:00 A.M., the child may continue asking, "What time is it now?" "How long till we leave?" "When is it going to be 3 o'clock?" It might be better for this parent to tell the child at 2:30, "Start getting dressed, we are going to Preston's birthday party." Another child's father tells him on Monday, "We are going to the football game Sunday," and the child is excited and wound up all week. The excitability might have been reduced if the father waited until Saturday to tell the child about the football game.

There is no standard answer about when to tell an overactive child about an upcoming event. It has to be done on an individual basis. You have to observe your child to determine what should be avoided and when you should tell him or her about an event in the future.

When excitable children are faced with a new situation and do not know what to expect, it is often helpful for the parent to try to make things as predictable as possible. This can primarily be accomplished by telling the child step by step what will happen. This could be the first day of baseball practice, a doctor's appointment, the child's first school fair, or whatever. By telling the child what may happen, you provide some structure and make the situation more predictable and less ambiguous.

Parents who have children with these characteristics can almost predict the situations where the children will become excited or moody. If this is the case, try to avoid these situations. Such situations may be playing with more than one child, long shopping trips, or some of the circumstances described above. Avoid winding a child up and then saying, "It's time to quit." For example, a father and his son may be wrestling. They are rolling around on the floor, tickling one another, and so on. Then the father says, "Let's stop" and they stop, but the child is wound up for the next hour. Try to engage in these interactions when it is all right for the child to remain excited (i.e., when he can go outside to play), and not when it's time to get ready for bed or when it is necessary to calm down.

Some parents tell me, "I know what kind of day it's going to be when she wakes up in the morning. I can tell if she's in a good or bad mood when she gets out of bed and comes in the kitchen." Try to recognize the child's "bad moods" and react to her differently or avoid things that will increase her excitability or moodiness. Other parents can identify when a child is getting wound up. That is, his behavior usually follows a sequence of events before he really gets excited. If you can tell when a child's excitability or moodiness is "building up," try to recognize it early to prevent it from getting out of hand. The child can be diverted to another activity, removed from the situation, or put in a time out area.

The above suggestions can be seen as preventive measures. Once a child becomes excited or gets in a "bad mood," other steps must be taken. Again, some parents have learned methods to calm down the excited child or to put her in a better mood. These techniques may involve removing the child from the situation, talking to her, using reward, or employing some of the suggestions discussed in Part II.

IMMEDIATE NEED SATISFACTION

Many overactive children are impatient. They want things *now*, not in five minutes or one hour. They have a difficult time with delays and find it hard to wait. Several things can be done to help a child develop patience or reduce the hassle that surrounds these behaviors.

Try to minimize waiting time. If you tell a child at 9:00 Saturday morning, "We are going to go to Grandma's house at 2:00," you are likely to hear every five minutes, "Is it 2:00 yet?" "When are we going to leave?" "I want to go now." Instead, at 1:30 you could tell him, "Start getting ready, we are going to Grandma's in a few minutes." Avoid giving the child long waiting periods. Tell him about events relatively close to when they are going to happen. Avoid statements like "Next Saturday we are going fishing." "Tomorrow you are going to Steven's birthday party."

Use cues in the environment to signify the end of the waiting period. For example, "When this TV program is over, we are going to get an ice cream." "When Momma comes home, we will go to the show." "As soon as the bell rings on the timer, you can go outside and play." By doing this, you often significantly reduce the child's questions.

If you know a child will have to wait (e.g., at the doctor's office, when his brother is playing a baseball game), give him something to do. Bring some toys, paper and pencil, a book, or anything else that may help him stay amused.

Positive consequences can also be used to help a child learn patience. Suppose you have a child who cannot wait ten minutes. At first, you may tell her two minutes before you are scheduled to leave the house. "We are leaving to go swimming in a few minutes. I am going to set the timer on the stove. If you do not ask me 'when are we going to leave' [explain exactly what you mean], we will stop and get a bag of potato chips on the way to the pool. If you ask me questions about when we will leave before the bell rings, we will not stop and get the chips." As the child is able to handle the delays successfully you would increase the time she has to wait before she receives the reward.

OPPOSITION

This behavior is usually a method of expressing anger or disapproval. If you are angry with me, it means that I am doing something you do not like. If your child shows aggressive or rebellious behaviors with you, his peers, or authority figures, it means that he disapproves of or does not agree with what other people are saying or doing. The anger could be expressed a variety of ways.

- She can express her feelings in an appropriate manner—"I don't like going to my room every time I do something bad. I wish you would stop doing that to me. It gets me angry when you do that to me."
- He could express his disapproval indirectly through passive-aggressive behaviors—stubbornness, sassiness, doing the opposite of what he is told.
- The child could acknowledge her anger directly by acting out her feelings physically—hitting or attempting to hit the person who she perceives as the source of her anger.
- He could displace his feelings to a less threatening person or to an inanimate object—the child may be angry with his mother, but he hits his sister, throws something, or breaks a toy. Some forms of dealing with anger will get the child in trouble; others will not.

METHODS OF EXPRESSING ANGER

Appropriate Communication

Appropriate communication involves the child telling the person who made him angry or with whom he disagrees how he feels. For example, his parent may holler at him, and he may say, "I don't like you hollering at me. That makes me feel bad." The child is expressing his feelings, and if this is done in a normal conversational tone and not in a sarcastic manner it is not sassiness. You should strive to have your children communicate their feelings. If they can express their anger without hollering or appearing sassy, "flip," or "smart", you should reinforce this and listen to them. It is not what is said, but how it is said. Some parents mistakenly view appropriate expression of feelings as disrespect or sassiness. The old saying, "A child should be seen and not heard" could not be further from the truth when talking about appropriate expressions of anger. You should want to hear what a child disapproves of or what makes her angry. This method of expressing anger will produce little, if any, problems for the child.

Passive-Aggressive Behaviors

Passive-aggressive behaviors are indirect ways of expressing anger. Suppose you go to work and your boss gives you a hard time first thing in the morning. She tells you what a bad job you are doing, that you may be fired, and similar things. In general, you are really angry at her, but you cannot punch her or quit the job. What will you do? You probably slow down your work. You may take a longer coffee break and may "forget" to do a few of the things she told you to do. You have passively acknowledged your anger in an attempt to retaliate.

Children frequently use this indirect method to express their anger. It usually takes the form of rebellion, doing the opposite of what is told, negativism, stubbornness, (you say "it's black" and the child says "it's white"), opposition, sassiness, mumbling, intentionally doing something he knows will aggravate, having the last word. For example, a child is sent to her room. She is angry, but what can she do? She starts mumbling, "You're unfair. You're always on my back, I want to live at Grandma's," and so forth. Her mother gets upset and starts hollering—the child has "gotten back" and has indirectly expressed her anger. This method of dealing with aggressive feelings is likely to produce problems in the child's relationships with others, especially those in a position of supervision or direction over her (i.e., parents and teachers).

Direct Acting Out of Anger

Direct acting out usually involves physical violence, fighting, or hitting. The child directly and physically retaliates against the source of his anger. For example, a boy will not give the child the football on the school playground, so he threatens to hit him or he starts a fight. This method of dealing with aggressive feelings will especially produce problems in peer interaction, but may also be seen in the child's relationships with authority.

Displacing Aggressive Feelings
Sometimes children become angry but do not deal directly with the source of their feelings. Instead they displace these emotions to a less threatening person or to an inanimate object. For example, a child's mother may do something that makes her angry. She does not say or do anything to her parent, but hits or aggravates her sister. A teacher reprimands a child in the cafeteria. She then leaves and the child starts pushing one of his classmates. A parent sends a child to her room for being sassy. While in her room, she breaks some of her toys. This method of dealing with anger is most likely to give the child problems in relationships with other children, peers, or siblings.

THE ANGER BALLOON

All children get angry, and these emotions are expressed in some fashion. Some methods of acknowledging aggressive feelings will produce problems; others will not. You can visualize this as an "anger balloon." Each time something happens that we do not like, it adds air to the balloon and it starts to expand. Air has to be let out of the balloon (i.e., anger has to be expressed) and the way this is done is different for different people. Some people let the anger build up until the balloon pops. When this happens, there may be an explosive outburst or a great deal of anger for a minor reason (the straw that broke the camel's back). After this display of anger, there is usually a period of control until the balloon blows up again. Other people release air out of the balloon every time it starts to fill up. These are the individuals who appropriately express their feelings at the time they occur. Other people release air through passive-aggressive maneuvers, displacement, or through their bodies (e.g., headaches).

When talking about dealing with aggressive and rebellious behaviors in children, we must consider three basic things: (1) how to help the child express and deal with anger, release the air from the balloon; (2) how to reduce the accumulation of anger or air in

the balloon; (3) how to deal with aggressive and oppositional behaviors when they occur.

MODELS

Parents serve as significant models for their children. The way we
handle conflicts and problems is apt to be imitated by our children.
If I handle my anger by being oppositional, stubborn, or punching
holes in the wall, there is a good probability that my children will
handle their conflicts similarly. The old saying "Don't do as I do,
do as I say" does not hold true. Therefore, if you are seeing aggressive or rebellious behaviors in your child, look at yourself and see if
you are modeling these. If you are, stop.

If there is a significant amount of hollering in the home and
adults do not respect one another, it is likely that their child will
also show these behavior patterns.

> One time a mother of a young sassy and stubborn child told me,
> "Every time I tell my child something, he says 'I'm not doing that,
> and if you don't like it pack your clothes and leave.' He's always
> putting me down. He shows no respect. It's like I'm the child and
> he's the parent." After some discussion, it was found out that this
> woman was treated in the same manner by her husband. Her child
> learned this behavior through modeling.
>
> Another mother told me, "Every time I hit my daughter, she hits me
> back. What should I do?" My answer was very simple, "Stop hitting
> her."

Whenever I see a child whose primary problem is fighting the first
question I ask the parents is, "How is he disciplined?" These children are usually dealt with through physical punishment or threats
of physical punishment. When we deal with children through
physical means, we are teaching them to handle conflicts or people
who do not comply with them by physical force or aggressive
behavior.

Parents must be sure they are not modeling the behaviors
they are trying to eliminate in their child. Serving as an appropriate
model is a good way to teach children how to deal with or express
their anger.

REDUCING THE BUILDUP OF ANGER

Avoid Random Discipline

Parents often discipline after the fact. They set a rule and wait till the child breaks it to decide on a consequence. With random disciplining, the child feels that you are responsible for what has happened to him, and anger is apt to develop.

Avoid Excessive Negative Attention

Negative consequences or punishment as the main method of control should be avoided. Eliminate verbal punishment (i.e., hollering, putting down a child, excessive criticism). Use reward as a disciplinary tactic. Emphasize the child's successes, accomplishments, and good behaviors. Pay more attention to "normal" good behaviors—when the child brushes his teeth after being told once, and so on.

DEALING WITH AGGRESSIVE AND REBELLIOUS BEHAVIOR

Even if these suggestions are implemented, stubbornness, fighting, opposition, and other behaviors that indicate underlying anger may be seen.

Use Positive Consequence

Avoid using violence to deal with violence. For example, a child hits his sister and gets a whipping. By using positive consequences, emphasis is placed on not fighting. "If you and your sister do not fight this afternoon, we will play that game you enjoy playing." Do not use force to deal with force. Behavior charts can also be used effectively to deal with some methods of expressing anger.

Ignore Passive-Aggressive Behaviors

Not only do children use passive-aggressive maneuvers to acknowledge anger, but they also employ these behaviors to get a reaction from their parents. Therefore, ignoring is often an effective way to reduce opposition, stubbornness, resistance, and similar behaviors.

In addition, the way parents often deal with passive-aggressive behavior results in a buildup of anger in the child. For example, a child asks her mother, "Can I stay up past my bedtime and finish watching this movie?" Her mother says, "no," and the child starts being sassy, making faces, and becoming defiant. These passive-aggressive behaviors are releasing anger and letting air out of her balloon. If the parent gets into a shouting match, more anger will develop and she will put more air into her child's anger balloon. The anger that is initially released by the sassiness is offset by a buildup of additional aggressive feelings. By using the consequence of ignoring, this additional buildup of anger can be eliminated.

NOT LISTENING, TEMPER TANTRUMS, AND SIMILAR BEHAVIORS

"Not listening" behaviors in overactive children are a very common problem. Parents often characterize their children as "hardheaded," "not doing what he is supposed to do," "unable to take 'No' for an answer." One of the reasons some of this behavior exists is inconsistency in the parent's methods of dealing with the child's behavior.

Another major cause of "not listening" behaviors in children is that parents often use verbal interaction as a method of discipline. For most children, this goes in one ear and comes out the other. A child sticks a pencil in his sister's ear and the parent says, "You know you shouldn't do that. You really make me upset when you and your sister fight. You may hurt her or make her deaf for the rest of her life. She's your sister and you should love her, you know how much she likes you," and so forth. This type of communication should be done, but do not expect talk to control or prevent behaviors. Ninety percent of the children I deal with will not be disciplined effectively with reasoning, talk, and verbal interchange, but will behave when consequences are employed. Talk should be restricted to conversation and *not* used as a disciplinary tactic. When verbal punishment is used to manage children, they often learn to be "parent deaf."

Another cluster of common behaviors ranges from severe

temper tantrums to silly facial expressions. These also include whining, pouting, crying, repeatedly asking similar questions or making statements (e.g., "Why can't I do it? Please let me go. Come on, give me one more chance"), complaining, silly noises, and similar actions. They occur for two reasons: either they get a reaction from the parent or they manipulate others so that the child will get her way.

When what this child is getting out of a behavior is "he's getting me upset, angry, or nervous," or "he's getting his way," then the consequence of ignoring should be employed. The parent should first withdraw all attention and consequences and deal with the behavior very matter-of-factly (see Chapter 6).

If ignoring is accurately employed and the behavior does not significantly change, then other consequences need to be tried. Regardless of the procedure employed, this type of behavior must be dealt with in a very calm manner, without any negative attention. A specific behavior chart could be set up using reward for appropriate behavior or response cost punishment.

chapter fourteen

POOR SELF-CONCEPT

Self-image and self-concept simply mean how you feel about yourself, how you see yourself compared to others. When a negative self-image exists, the child sees himself as made up of more negative qualities than positive traits, and numerous other problems are apt to emerge. This usually develops when more emphasis is placed on a child's faults, failures, and misbehaviors than on her successes and accomplishments.

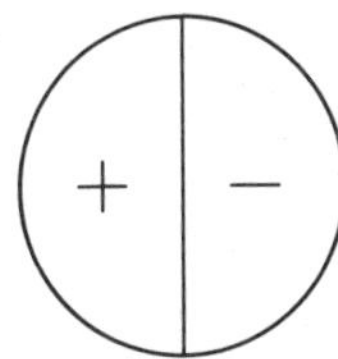

Figure 14.1. Original Self-Concept

Suppose the circle in Figure 14-1 represents our personality when we are born. Half is composed of positive qualities—things we can do as well as or better than other people. The other half is composed of negative qualities or skills—things we cannot do so well or things other people can do better. Let's say that you can cook—that would fall on the plus side. I cannot cook, so in my circle this skill would fall on the minus side. However, I know something about refinishing furniture, and that would fall on the plus side of my circle. You do not know anything about this, so for you this skill would be a minus. The point is: although you have a lot of skills superior to mine, I have an equal amount that I can do as well as or better than you. Therefore, when we look at the overall picture, we are basically the same in terms of our value and competence. What makes us different is that we have different skills in different areas. The same situation exists for children.

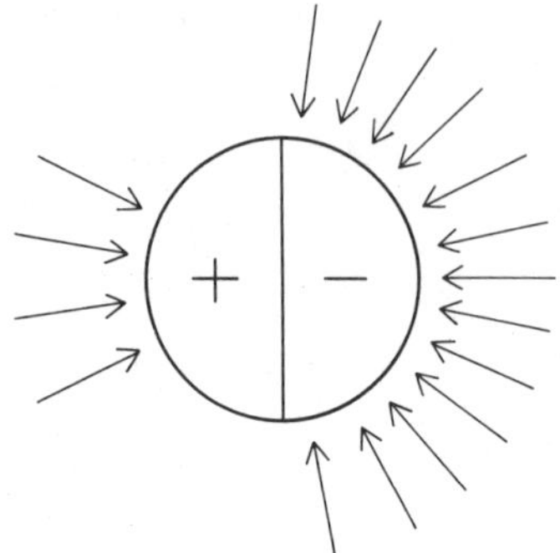

Figure 14.2. Effect of Negative Attention on Self-Image

However, when more emphasis is placed on negative traits than on the positive side (see Figure 14-2), a negative self-image starts to develop. The overactive child is frequently faced with this situation. Suppose two children come to your house. One has overactive characteristics and the other does not. You can bet that the overactive child will have to be corrected (e.g., "don't touch that," "keep still") much more frequently than the child without these behavioral aspects. Children with overactive characteristics generally receive a significant amount of negative attention because their behavior often does not conform to what is expected. A negative self-image can also develop if more attention is paid to a child's misbehavior than to his appropriate actions. Suppose a child does fifty things in a day. Twenty-five are good and twenty-five are bad. The child usually gets attention for two of the twenty-five good behaviors, and emphasis is placed on twenty-four of the twenty-five bad ones. Good behaviors are overlooked because they are expected. If the child is doing what he is supposed to, nobody says anything but let him rock the boat and we are quick to notice. For example, the child is supposed to make his bed. He makes it six days but forgets to make it the seventh day. Parents usually give attention for bed-making behavior on the day the child fails to make the bed.

This excessive negative attention can also build up when a lot of punishment is used on a child. Negative consequences tend to place emphasis on "bad" behavior and overlook "good" behaviors. For example, a parent may tell a child, "I want you home by 5:00. If you're late you won't be able to look at TV tonight." Now, the child comes in late and gets a lecture, punishment, and a great deal of attention for this misbehavior. Probably the only thing that would have happened if he did come home on time is that he would not have gotten punished.

If expectations exceed capabilities, if a parent expects a child to get *A*s and *B*s, but she is of average intelligence and her best is represented by *C*s, then she will be failing much more frequently than she is succeeding. Some people also expect a six-year-old child to act like he is twelve years old. If behavioral or performance expectations are set above the child's capabilities, he is certain to experience failure and unnecessary negative attention. Overactive children who have school difficulties receive more negative attention than other children. Students who have trouble with their schoolwork experience frustration, failure, and emphasis on their negative traits much more often than those children who have few academic problems. This negative attention comes not only from school but also from home. Most parents tend to put more "pressure" or attention on the child's failures at school if she is having trouble there.

Regardless of the origin of negative emphasis, certain personality changes may occur in overactive children who receive more attention to their failures than to their successes and accomplishments. The most dramatic can be seen in Figure 14-3.

There is a gradual change in how the child sees himself. The positive side starts decreasing, with a corresponding increase on the negative side. He tends to view himself as being made up of more failures, mistakes, and weak points than successes, accom-

Figure 14.3. Development of Negative Self-Image

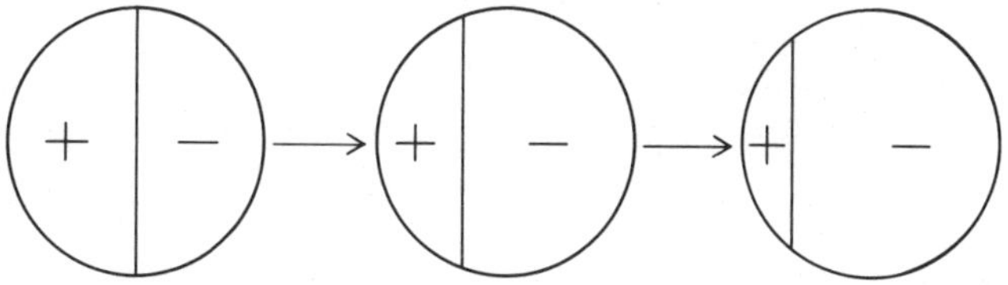

plishments, and achievements. He sees his peers as being more capable, effective, and competent than he, and he generally lacks pride in himself.

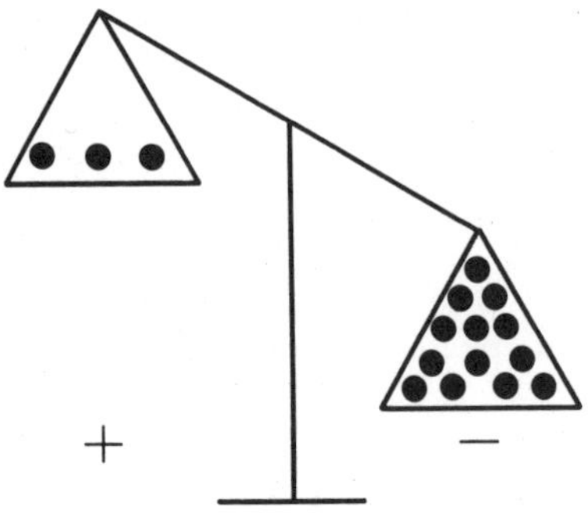

Figure 14.4. The Self-Image Scale

If we see this as a scale (Figure 14-4), the child perceives the negative side as having a very large pile of rocks, while the positive side of the scale has very few. Once the scale gets off balance (a negative image develops), something has to be done to get it back to a balanced position.

THE CHILD'S ATTEMPT TO DEAL WITH A POOR SELF-CONCEPT

One way the child with a poor self-image attempts to get his scales balanced is to avoid getting any more rocks on the negative side. He will avoid any situation that may produce failure, frustration, or criticism or any situation that accentuates his weak points. Therefore, he may avoid competition or any win-loss situation. If he does compete, he will not be able to stand coming in second and usually will be a poor loser. If the child with a poor self-image starts something and it gets difficult, she will give up easily. In addition, she would much rather not try something than to try it and fail. Such a child does not like new situations and will tend to avoid going places or doing things where he is not sure of himself. We usually interpret the above behaviors as a lack of confidence.

If you punish, criticize, reprimand, or otherwise stress a weak point, a child with a poor self-concept will often react significantly.

You may not mean anything by your comments, but they provoke a reaction. Let's say a child is putting a model together, but is going about it the wrong way. You very calmly say, "Why not do it this way? It will be easier." The child reacts violently because he reads what you said as "I'm screwing up again." It is as if another rock is placed on his negative side. This is when you see sensitivity, pouting, temper tantrums, or similar behaviors, depending on the personality of the child.

We all look for things in the environment that support the way we feel about ourselves. A child with a negative self-image will look for things that support his feelings. He may be hypersensitive to things that he views as negative. For example, a child may raise his hand in class to answer a question, but the teacher calls on someone else. The child with a negative image may feel that the teacher does not like him.

In addition to avoiding situations that produce negative attention, the child can balance the scales by seeking out situations that produce positive attention, that is, trying to pile rocks on the plus side of the scale. The child will gravitate toward experiences where she has success, gets pats on the back, or feels a sense of accomplishment. Let's say a child helps his mother bake a cake. Some neighbors come over, tell the child how good it is, and give him a lot of positive attention. The next several days he may be asking to help his mother bake another cake. Another example would be a child who writes a note telling her parents how much she loves them. Her mother and father get the note and hug and kiss her. For the next six days these parents will be receiving many similar notes. Children want to engage in behaviors that will get them positive attention.

To get positive attention children may also develop inappropriate or "bad" behaviors, such as being the class clown, constantly demanding attention and approval from the teacher, or getting involved with an unacceptable peer group because they feel comfortable with this group of kids.

HOW A POOR SELF-CONCEPT MAY BE EXPRESSED

The child, depending on his or her personality, may adopt one or a combination of the behavioral styles below to deal with a negative self-concept.

Accepting What He or She Feels
The Environment Is Saying

If the child feels as if he is trying his best but it is not good enough, he may accept what he feels the environment is telling him. "I'm trying my best, but I still don't know what's happening and I'm getting more and more negative attention. There must be something wrong with me. Maybe I am useless, bad, and inferior to others." If your faults are pointed out frequently enough, you begin thinking you have an excessive number of them and start acting in that fashion.

Such children are often shy, somewhat withdrawn, and show an obvious lack of confidence. They tend to belittle themselves and may appear unhappy and dissatisfied.

Masking Inadequacies

Another way children deal with a negative self-image is to try to mask their inadequacies, and present a front showing just positive qualities. For example, a child would communicate to others that she is the greatest: "I have the best house, I never make mistakes, I'm never wrong." However, that child is actually telling you that she feels she has numerous faults, but she is not going to let you see any of them, because if you see one you will see what a bad person she is and will not like her.

Children often respond in this manner when a negative self-image is present. They do not admit to mistakes and do not accept responsibility for their own behavior. Someone else is always at fault, they quickly blame others for their mistakes, and they always have a string of excuses to explain their behavior.

Developing a Pleasure Orientation

A third method children use to deal with a poor self-image is to "tune out" the environment and become more concerned with their needs and wishes than the wants, desires, and rules of others. Some children respond as if they are thinking, "I don't know what I have to do to get positive attention or to please other people, so the heck with them. But I do know what I have to do to please me or to make me happy, so I'm going to do that."

In this situation you get a "pleasure-oriented" child. The child is primarily concerned with satisfying his own needs and wishes. He is more concerned with the pleasure he derives from his behavior than the punishment.

Although they can be polite, charming, and affable when it is to their advantage, these children generally have problems with authority or those in a position of supervision or direction over them. They often are rebellious, stubborn, oppositional, and resistant. In school, a variety of problems are often seen in such children and are usually characterized by an inability to follow classroom procedure. It looks as if this child has not developed any internal control, self-discipline, or responsibility because she does what she pleases when she pleases.

Because of the pleasure orientation, punishment does not work well, often not at all, with this type of child. Negative consequences, when they do work, only affect this type of child temporarily—for a few minutes, at best a few days. Therefore, reward has to be primarily used in dealing with these children.

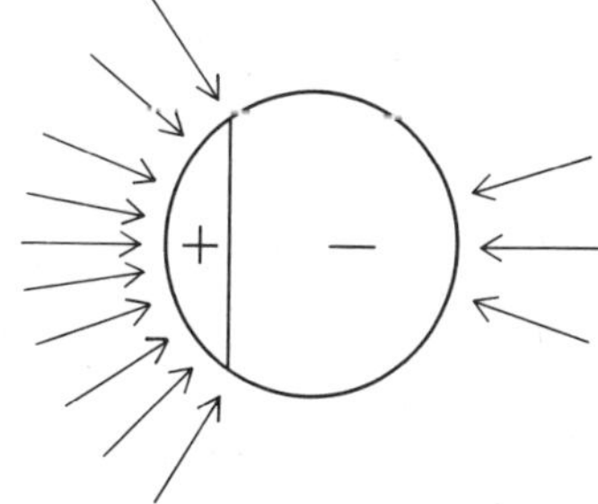

Figure 14.5. Improving Poor Self-Image

CHANGING A POOR SELF-IMAGE
AND BUILDING CONFIDENCE

To eliminate a negative self-concept, build confidence, and make the child feel better about himself, you have to reverse the process that produced the poor self-image (see Figure 14-5). More attention must be given to the child's successes, accomplishments, and positive personality characteristics than to his failures, mistakes, and misbehaviors. When this starts happening the plus side of the personality begins to increase, with a corresponding decrease on the negative, and the child's self-confidence starts improving. There are several ways this can be accomplished.

Using Reward as the Primary Disciplinary Tactic

Often when I tell parents they have to take the emphasis off what a child is doing wrong and place it on to what she is doing right, they misinterpret it as not disciplining the child. To the contrary, the overactive child needs a lot of structure. However, negative consequences should be minimized and reward should be emphasized.

Attending to Everyday Positive Behaviors

Sometimes when I tell parents that we want to strengthen the child's self-image I am told, "We already do that. When he brings home a good grade, hits a home run, or wins the science fair, we praise him." These parents are saying that any time something *major* happens the child gets positive attention. How often do these things happen?—once a week, twice a month, three times a year. On the other hand, how many interactions do you have with your child daily? If the majority of these are negative, positive things that happen once a week or twice a month are not going to offset this negative buildup. Although we want to attend to the child's major successes, we can accomplish much more by paying attention to his daily "good" behaviors, because they occur more frequently.

Look for daily good behaviors and praise the child for these. They may be making her bed, going to bed when told, saying "thank you," or whatever. By looking at these behaviors, you can increase the amount of positive attention the child is receiving each day, and this will produce change.

Placing Realistic Expectations on the Child

Behavioral and performance expectations should be in line with the child's capabilities so that he can experience success, approval, and other forms of positive attention.

Overlooking Some Overactive Behaviors

To reduce the negative attention for some children, parents have to take a general look at the types of overactive behaviors and rank them in the order of importance. Some of the "less important" overactive behaviors can then be overlooked.

chapter fifteen

PEER CONFLICT

Because of their impulsiveness, inability to concentrate, short attention span, and other behaviors, overactive children often have difficulty relating to other children. However, their "bossy" and "domineering" attitude is often the primary reason for the difficulties in their relationships with other children. They need to be the leader, take control, and tell everybody else what to do. This attitude may be an attempt for the child to structure the environment and make it more predictable. If he is in control and "calling the shots," then he knows what will happen. However, if another child is in control and setting the rules, the situation is less structured. Conflict, fighting, and arguing usually occur when one child tries to take control, and this is often followed by rejection from other children.

Bossing behavior is more intense when the child is playing with more than one playmate. That is, some overactive children play well with one child, but add one, two, or three more and problems develop. Therefore, one way to reduce these peer problems is to restrict the number of children he plays with to one at a time. Introduce other children gradually, using reward and the techniques described in Part II. For example, if the child has been playing well with one child, you could then have him play with two children for short periods of time. He could be told, "You can have Alan and Glen over to play for a little while [depending on the child's age, it would be ten to thirty minutes]. If you can get along with them [explain exactly what you mean by this] for several minutes, we'll take a ride and get some popcorn." The length of time that you allow the child to play with more than one child could be gradually increased as he is able to play successfully without conflict. A time out form of punishment could also be used in this situation. "Alan and Glen are coming over to play. Whenever I hear you fighting with them, you will have to come inside for five minutes."

Some overactive children cannot avoid conflicts when they play over long periods of time with other children. They may be able to play fine with another child for thirty to forty-five minutes, but after that they are almost certain to have difficulties. If your child shows this pattern, simply limit her play periods to the length of time she can handle. Two forty-five-minute play periods with a half-hour break may produce significantly fewer problems than one hour-and-a-half play period. To determine how long a play period should be, you have to look at the individual child and see if there is any pattern to her conflicts.

Because overactive children often experience conflict with children their own age, they may gravitate toward playmates younger or older than they. If the majority of their play involves children significantly different in age, other problems are certain to arise. For example, if a nine or ten year old primarily plays with five and six year olds, he is probably dominating the play and learning immature methods of interacting with others. With children his own age he may feel uncomfortable and out of place, or the skills he has learned may cause him to be rejected by his peers. Therefore, it is important that the majority of your child's play be with children his own age so that he can learn age-appropriate skills. Often when I tell parents this, they say, "She's in school all day with children her age." That may be true, but in her six- or seven-hour school day, she is probably only playing with others for twenty-five to thirty minutes during recess and lunch. A child having socialization difficulties may need more contact with children her age than she gets in school.

Frequently the conflict seen in the overactive child's play is not confined to her peers. It may also involve her brothers and sisters. When fighting and conflict involve the child's siblings, some of the general management techniques in Part II and the section in Chapter 13 on opposition can be used.

Another technique to reduce sibling conflict is to look at the child's primary playmate. Suppose two brothers close in age, Jason and Alan, are constantly fighting. You would ask, ''Who is Jason's primary playmate?'' (the child he plays with the majority of the time). If the answer is Alan, you would try to get them different primary playmates. Have a child come over after school, invite a child over on Saturday, or whatever. Often this simple move will significantly reduce the conflict between the brothers.

chapter sixteen
SCHOOL PROBLEMS

Some parents are happy to have the summer end so the kids will be back in school. However, others dread the end of summer because school means teacher conferences, grades, and homework. For these parents the start of school brings arguing, fighting, and repeated attempts to have their child do homework, study for a test, make adequate grades, and behave in class. This chapter will discuss methods to deal with school-related concerns.

GRADES

Parents make several general mistakes concerning grades and school performance. One is that they expect too much from some children. For half of the children in the United States, "doing their best" or performing at their potential means average or C work. However, some parents view a C as an unacceptable grade and demand As and Bs. When expectations for a child's performance are higher than his capabilities, we are almost assuring that he will fail. If school becomes a negative experience, the child is apt to avoid it and start to show a lack of interest.

Another general mistake that parents make is attempting to deal with or improve their child's grades over too long a period of time. Most schools have grading periods of six to nine weeks, and often disciplinary measures are put into effect "till the next report card." For most children this is too long, and several problems are apt to arise.

Let's say a child has failed two subjects because he was not prepared for tests and had not been turning in the required work. His parents tell him, "You will have to spend two hours in your room each day doing your homework and studying, and you will not be allowed to go outside and play until your grades improve." Now, if this means till the next report card, or four and one half weeks till the progress reports are issued, several things may occur. First, this child will probably sit in his room each day and do anything other than studying. Second, when long punishments are used to improve grades, two typical patterns occur. Some children work hard in the beginning, about one or two weeks, but because there is no immediate payoff, go back to their old ways and their grades do not improve. Other children fool around during most of the punishment and work hard the last week or two before the report card. However, this last-minute burst of studying does not improve their overall grades and they continue to be punished. They are actually punished for working hard because of the principle of immediacy of consequences.

When working with grades, it is best to set short-term goals—on a daily or weekly basis. When I am working with a family where grades are a concern I usually tell the parents, "Forget about the grades, and let's look at his behavior." What I mean is that you have to look at what the child is doing that is resulting in the poor grades. For example, let's say you get your child's report card and she has failed math. The first question to ask is, "Why has she failed?" This can usually be answered by having a meeting with her teacher. You find out that she has done poorly because she has not been turning in her homework or completing her math seat work. Now that you have the reason for her poor performance, you can focus on this. Rather than saying "till your grades improve," you would say "till your behavior [or the reasons] for the poor grades improves." If the reason a child has done poorly in a subject is he has not done his homework and class assignments, you can safely assume that if you can change this, his grades will also change.

Administer consequences on a daily or weekly basis. For

example, "Each day you complete your seat work and turn in your homework, you can stay up past your bedtime" or "if you complete your seat work and turn in your homework four out of five times this week, we will go fishing Saturday." The parent would have to establish a communication system with the school and could use a behavior chart or one of the other techniques described in Chapter 10. If you can get the child to turn in all his homework and complete his seat work on a daily basis, his grades will show an improvement at the end of the nine-week period.

BRINGING HOME ASSIGNMENTS

Children learn very rapidly that if they do not write all of the assignment they will have to spend less time on their homework, if they "forget" a book in school they will not have to study that subject, or if they "lose" a bad test paper or note from the teacher they will not get punished.

A common statement by parents is, "The teacher says he's doing poorly because he's not prepared for class and is not doing all his homework. But I don't know what he has to study or what he has for homework, or he tells me he finished it at school." There are several ways to deal with this situation. First, some communication system must be established between the parent and school. Next, get the child an assignment book and have him record all the assignments. At the end of the period or day, he brings the book to the teacher and he or she initials *through* the assignment (see Figure 16-1).

This procedure only requires a few seconds of the teacher's time. You would make the child responsible for getting the signature. In addition, you could set up appropriate consequences for bringing or not bringing the assignment home signed. For example, on the days it is brought home signed he earns extra play time, TV time, or whatever. When it is not brought home signed, there could be negative consequences.

If a child keeps telling you she completed a certain assignment in school, set up a general rule that you have to see all completed work. If something is left in school, she will have to do it again at home.

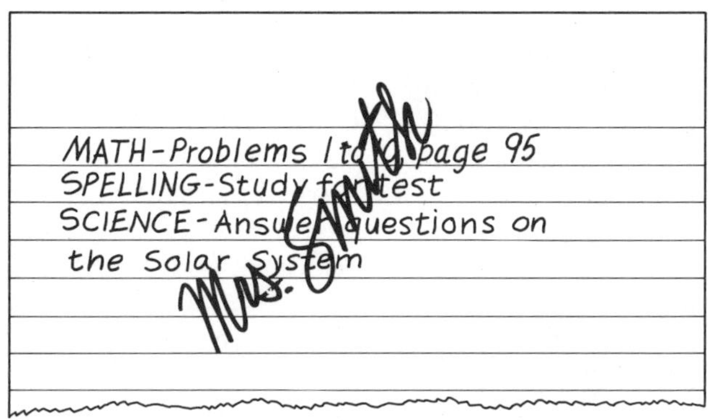

Figure 16.1. Monday's Assignment

During the past school year I got a call from my oldest son's teacher informing me that he was doing poorly in math. It was a surprise, and I asked the teacher, "How can that be? He's getting good grades on his tests." The teacher told me that this was not true—he had failed about half of the math tests he had taken that grading period. However, I had not seen them. When I questioned my son, he said that he had "lost" them or had put them in his desk drawer and "forgot" to tell us about them. Because we were not seeing the bad test papers, we did not know of his poor performance or that he needed help in certain areas. We then set up a behavior chart on which he earned points for *every* math test brought home. He received more points for passing grades than failing ones, but he was not given a great deal of negative attention for the bad test papers. Soon we were seeing all of the test papers and then could identify his weak areas and give extra help.

The main reason for a child "forgetting" or "losing" tests is to avoid negative attention or punishment. Therefore, you should try to deal with these behaviors by using positive consequences. Not remembering to bring home books, a coat, or whatever could be dealt with in a similar fashion.

HOMEWORK

Getting children to do their homework seems to be a never-ending battle for most parents. Some of the techniques mentioned above may ease this problem. A question I am frequently asked is, "When should I have my child do his homework? As soon as he comes from school, or should I let him have a break or play first?" There is no pat answer to this question. Some children can go out and play and then come in and do the required work; other children, if you allow them to play first, are harder to get back in or calmed down to actually do the homework. Parents should use the method that works most appropriately with their child. However, a general procedure is to establish a routine or have a certain time each day when homework is done (e.g., after school, after dinner, before watching TV at night, 5:00). Children who have a set time to do homework generally give less problems than those who do not.

The overactive child with a short attention span may have particular difficulty with homework. For these children it is best to break up the homework period. In addition, they need a quiet place, free from distraction, to do their homework.

Some children try to avoid homework because they receive a great deal of negative attention at that time. Homework time for some kids means that parents get upset, so children try everything in their power to prevent this. Most parents become too upset and frustrated when helping their child with schoolwork. This is the main reason parents do not make good tutors, even if they are teachers. Although it is easier said than done, you should try to deal with homework in a very calm, matter-of-fact way and reduce the amount of negative attention the child receives. Deal with the child and his behaviors in this situation positively. Set up expectations and consequences as outlined in Chapter 3.

Natural Consequences
Some behaviors carry their own consequences.

"Go do your homework. It should take a half hour to complete if you apply yourself, but if you fool around it will take three hours, and that will mean that you will have less play time."

"Your sister and I are going to your grandmother's house at 7:00. If you finish your homework by that time, you can come with us. If you are not finished, you will have to stay home with your father and finish it."

Grandma's Rule
You do what I want you to do, then you can do what you want to do.

"You can't go outside and play until the homework is finished."

"You can watch TV when you complete your work."

Arbitrarily Set Consequences

Set expectations for the child using a consequence that is important to her.

"If you do your homework without giving me a hassle, you can stay up past your bedtime. If you give me trouble, you will go to bed at the regular time."

"If you finish your homework by 7:00 three out of the next four nights, Saturday we will go get those handle grips for your bike you have been wanting. If you do not, we'll just try it again next week."

Some parents must sit with their children the entire time to get the homework done. If they are not physically close to their children, nothing happens. Although it is good for parents to help their children with their homework, it is not necessary for the child to become excessively dependent on the parent to accomplish this task. The procedures above can be used to make the child more independent when it comes to doing homework. In some instances, the behavior (sitting with the child) you are trying to eliminate can serve as the reward. For example, you have to sit with your child for him to do ten math problems for homework. However, you tell him, "I have something to do. You do the first two by yourself and then I will sit with you to do the rest of them." After a week you could require the child to do three or four math problems before sitting with him. The number would then be gradually increased.

REFUSING TO ATTEND SCHOOL

Most children are not thrilled about going to school, but some show extreme reactions—crying, fears, physical complaints, refusal to separate from their parent—to avoid attending school. This usually happens in three general situations: when the child first starts school, when there have been significant changes in the child's environment, or when the child is experiencing problems in school.

Some children, especially those who have been dependent on their mother or who have not played or interacted with many children, often show this problem when they enter kindergarten or first grade. The primary remedy is to have the child remain at school. Teachers are aware of this problem and use various methods to deal with it in the classroom. Crying, temper tantrums, and so on are usually more intense when the parent is present, so you should try to get the child to school, treat the behaviors in a very matter-of-fact manner, and leave. A reward could also be used in this situation. It is also helpful if parents try to develop more independent behaviors in the home, to have the child play more with children his or her age, and to promote friendships with children in the child's class. The child in this situation wants to avoid school because of the newness of the situation and a feeling that he cannot function apart from his parent. Once he becomes used to the environment and gains more confidence in his ability to function alone in the classroom, the problem usually diminishes. However, if the parent continually brings the child home because she is upset or allows her to miss school frequently, a more intense problem is apt to develop and remain with the child throughout the elementary-school years.

Some children who experience significant change in their environment develop problems relating to attending school. They show fears or anxiety in the academic setting, general nervousness, or an inability to separate from their mother that make it difficult for them to remain in the classroom or building. The change could be a move, new school, divorce, remarriage, or death of a close relative. Again, it is important to keep the child in school rather than to let him stay home "to get over it." Although the child in this situation usually appears very upset, it is best to deal with the behavior very calmly and avoid excessive punishment, threats, and hollering. This child usually avoids attending school not because of something there but because he fears separating from his parent, usually his mother, and has general feelings of insecurity in his environment. Therefore, this type of problem must be dealt with indirectly through changes at home. Behavior charts and positive consequences can also be employed. Children with these problems are usually good students who do not show behavioral problems at school.

Other children refuse to attend school because they are experiencing problems in the academic setting. They are having academic or behavioral difficulties, and school has become a negative experience to be avoided. Although these children may show some of the behaviors described above, they typically use physical complaints to stay home, skip school, or have numerous "excuses" for not wishing to go to school (e.g., the teacher talks too fast, the child next to me keeps bothering me). It is best to get an evaluation to identify the source of this problem. Many times children who show this pattern have a learning problem. Once it is identified and steps are made to remedy the learning deficit, refusal to attend school diminishes.

ACADEMIC DIFFICULTIES

Some overactive children have problems with schoolwork because of their short attention span, distractibility, increased activity level, and so on. Other children show learning difficulties in addition to the characteristics of overactivity and require individual instruction or special education services. Tutoring may help some of these children, but the majority require changes in the school setting (see Chapter 10).

Some overactive children have academic difficulties because of perceptual-motor or visual-motor problems (see Chapter 17).

HOW TO COUNTER
NEGATIVE ATTENTION

Children attend school about half of the time they are awake. If you add homework, class projects, and related activities to this, school probably involves 60 percent to 70 percent of a child's life. When children are having trouble in school, a large portion of their lives involves negative attention. Therefore, it is very important that parents provide positive attention. In fact, these children should receive much more positive attention at home than children who are not experiencing difficulty at school to offset the excessive negative attention.

chapter seventeen

PERCEPTUAL-MOTOR DEFICITS

Some overactive children experience fine- or gross-motor coordination problems. Deficits in fine-motor coordination are also termed *perceptual-motor* or *visual-motor problems*. Because these difficulties occur much more frequently than deficits in gross-motor functioning, the majority of the chapter will be devoted to perceptual-motor deficits.

Gross-motor coordination refers to skills and abilities we normally think about in terms of coordination—riding a bike, jumping a rope, playing sports. When a child has problems in this area, he is usually described as poorly coordinated or clumsy. Although this deficit does not interfere with the child's ability to perform academically, it often produces social problems, especially for boys. These children have difficulty with sports and are usually picked last when sides are formed for a team game. They are usually seen as poor athletes and are often criticized. Therefore, problems in this area usually produce socialization difficulties and negative attention from the child's peers.

Perceptual-motor or *visual-motor deficits* refer to problems in fine-motor or hand-eye coordination. This pertains to how well the child's eyes and hands work together or how well she can reproduce with her hands what she sees. Children experiencing difficulties in these areas have trouble with paper-and-pencil tasks.

As youngsters, children with visual-motor problems often

stay away from paper-and-pencil tasks. They do not like to color, draw, cut and paste, or practice their ABCs. Handwriting requires a great deal of energy and effort. In their early school years these children have difficulty completing seat work, their penmanship or coloring is poor, their work is sloppy and disorganized. These children often reverse or invert letters and numbers and sometimes write words or their names backward. They have trouble copying from the board because they lose their place or leave out letters, words, or whole phrases. Sometimes they confuse letters, *d*s are called *b*s and *w*s are pronounced *m*, and confuse or read words backward, *saw* is read as *was* or *felt* is pronounced *left*.

The majority of kindergarten children reverse letters and numbers or write them backward. Therefore, such problems in kindergarten should not be a concern. About 50 percent of beginning first graders show reversals, but only about 10 percent of beginning second graders have problems in this area. Consequently, if the characteristics of perceptual-motor deficits are seen at this grade level, there is a strong probability that the child has problems in this area.

The child who has perceptual-motor problems does not necessarily have poor vision. The trouble is not in eyes or hands, but in processing what the eyes see. The problem lies in translating the information through the brain from eyes to hands. It is good, though, to get a vision exam. In fact, all children in their early school years should have their eyes checked once a year.

Perceptual-motor problems usually occur in two types of overactive children—those whose increased levels of activity result from a hyperkinetic reaction of childhood or those who have a depressed level of intelligence.

HYPERACTIVITY

Perceptual-motor deficits seen in hyperactive children usually result from a developmental deviation or lag. A child may be seven years old but shows the visual-motor development of a five year old. These deficits will improve with age. Around puberty, when all skills level out, the visual-motor problems will often diminish.

Perceptual-motor deficits resulting from lags in development can sometimes be improved with training. Some medical centers, universities, or hospitals in your community may have perceptual-motor training programs. Sometimes this training can be obtained privately. Children enrolled in these programs usually go for thirty to sixty minutes two or three times a week. They engage in activities to build perceptual-motor skills, and usually their parents are given activities to do with them at home.

Generally, parents can try to gear the child's play toward activities that will strengthen these skills. Toys that require hand-eye coordination skills can be purchased. A store that has educational supplies for teachers usually has a variety of games and activities to enhance perceptual-motor abilities. The lists below, prepared by Mallary Collins, M.Ed., will give you some ideas.

Fine Motor Activities
1. Tracing, coloring, cutting, pasting
2. Dot-to-dot sheets, puzzles, finger painting
3. Lacing boards, weaving games
4. Building models, clay
5. Jacks, Pick-up sticks, puppets
6. Building blocks, Lincoln Logs, Tinker Toys, Erector sets, Legos
7. Buttoning, unbuttoning, tying, zipping
8. Some electronic video games (e.g., baseball, Atari)

If a child has poor penmanship, it is better to have her practice paper-and-pencil tasks that she enjoys (e.g., coloring, tracing) than to have her excessively practice her penmanship. While most children who show perceptual-motor deficits do not necessarily have gross-motor coordination problems, practice in this area does seem indirectly to improve fine-motor skills. The activities below will be beneficial for children experiencing gross- and/or fine-motor coordination difficulties.

It is important for parents to remember that a child with motor impairments will appear clumsy and awkward. He may also appear disoriented. This is usually because he has not developed laterality and left-right perception. The child must learn to move his body in an organized fashion through space. To accomplish this, the following activities can be used.

The activities in the following list are easily done and require no specialized materials.

Gross Motor Activities

1. Walking Activities. Have the child walk in various ways—forward, backward, sideways. The child could also imitate various animals—elephant, duck, crab.
2. Crawling Activities. Have the child crawl imitating various activities—move like a snake, worm, or soldier.
3. Walking Hockey. Have the child move an object across the floor with his feet to a goal. Use points and play with teams.
4. Obstacle Course. Arrange an obstacle course using chairs, tables, boxes, and other objects. Have the child move through the course in a variety of ways.
5. Balance Beam. Use a 2' × 4' placed on the floor. Have the child move on it in different directions.
6. Exercises. Any exercise is good—jumping jacks, hopping, bending.
7. Dodge ball, leap frog
8. Simon says, hokeypokey
9. Ball games—throwing, catching, and kicking activities. These do not necessarily include organized sports. The child with motor problems should not be forced into organized sports until he or she wants to participate.
10. Bike riding, roller skating, skateboarding, hopscotch

DEPRESSED LEVEL OF INTELLIGENCE

The characteristics of overactivity, as well as perceptual-motor deficits, seen in these children usually result from organic or brain damage. Their hand-eye coordination difficulties do not improve with age. Therefore, these children may make some improvement using the above activities, but generally their visual-motor deficits will not show significant change with practice. Parents of these children may have to accept their difficulties and attempt to work around them. However, training should be attempted to help the child achieve his or her maximum potential.

Some children with perceptual-motor problems have learning disabilities, however, the majority will only have difficulty with handwriting activities. Because much of the work in the elementary grades involves paper-and-pencil tasks, their performance is frequently inadequate. The teacher needs to give such children individual consideration. Instead of marking the math problem or spelling word wrong when it is obvious the child has reversed some part of it, the teacher should ask him to spell the word orally, watch her do the math problem, or use some other method to see if the child knows the correct method. His penmanship should not be compared to that of others, and if the child is trying her best, she should be graded accordingly. The child may be slow writing and may require extra time to do seat work or he may need to be graded on what he has completed. For example, a teacher gives the class ten questions and the students have to write the answers. The child with perceptual-motor difficulties only finishes six although he tried hard, did not fool around, and put forth a 100 percent effort. If this is the case, he should be graded on the six completed and not receive a failing grade because he did not get to four of the questions. These children may have to be given less written homework and more verbal work to do. Other considerations may also have to be taken depending on the specific difficulties of the child.

chapter eighteen
CONCLUSION

I hope the information in this book has given you a better understanding of your overactive child and provided you with some alternate methods to deal with him or her on a daily basis. You still may have many questions regarding your child's behavior. If this is the case, contact your child's doctor or a mental health professional who deals with children.

Throughout the book I have mentioned that the methods described in the sections on General Management Techniques can be used on all types of overactivity. An effective behavior management system, as well as consistent discipline and the use of rewards, should be implemented in the home before more specific techniques of management are tried. Medication should be the last resort, used only after other techniques are not successful.

INDEX

! WORKSHOPS ON MANAGING CHILD BEHAVIOR !

For information on types of workshops, convention pre-
sentations, inservice training seminars, etc., contact
the author directly at either of the following addresses:

Dr. Don H. Fontenelle
St. Bernard Developmental Center
3114 Paris Road
Chalmette, LA 70043
Phone: 504-279-5427

or

Dr. Don H. Fontenelle
St. Bernard Developmental Center
118 Ridgelake Drive
Metairie, LA 70001
Phone: 504-831-3101

! FREE CATALOG !

Send for free catalog of Innovative Curriculum Guide-
books And Materials in MOVEMENT EDUCATION, SPE-
CIAL EDUCATION, and PERCEPTUAL-MOTOR DE-
VELOPMENT. Write:

FRONT ROW EXPERIENCE
540 Discovery Bay Blvd.
Byron, CA 94514
Questions? Call 415-634-5710